Indian Medical Science Series No. 129

Ayurveda *for* Child Health Care

Prof. Dr. P.H. Kulkarni

Sri Satguru Publications
A Division of
Indian Books Centre
Delhi - India

Published by
Sri Satguru Publications,
Indological and Ayurvedic Publishers
A Division of
Indian Books Centre
40/5, Shakti Nagar,
Delhi-110007
India

Email: ibcindia@vsnl.com
Website: http://www.indianbookscentre.com

First Edition; Pune,2000

Second Edition : Delhi , 2002

ISBN 81-7030-734-1

Published by Sunil Gupta for Sri Satguru Publications, a division of Indian Books Centre, 40/5, Shakti Nagar, Delhi-110007, India and printed at Chawla Offset Printers, Delhi 110 052

This book is Dedicated to

Persons needs Effective

Ayurvedic advise for

needy Children

all over the world

Prof. Dr. P. H. Kulkarni

FOREWORD

Embryo, Foetus transforms into Child and ultimately adult humanbeing.

Information bout development, influence of environment, role of Doshas, in the formation and development of living human is very important.

This information helps for preserving health of a Child, preventive measures and methods for cure of ailments.

Ayurveda offers many aspects in the development of Child. This information is useful for all and everywhere.

Prod. Dr. P. H. Kulkarni

Paris
France
December, 2000

INDEX

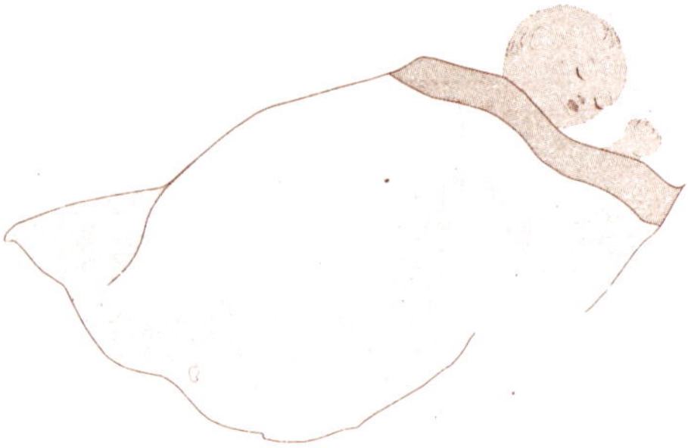

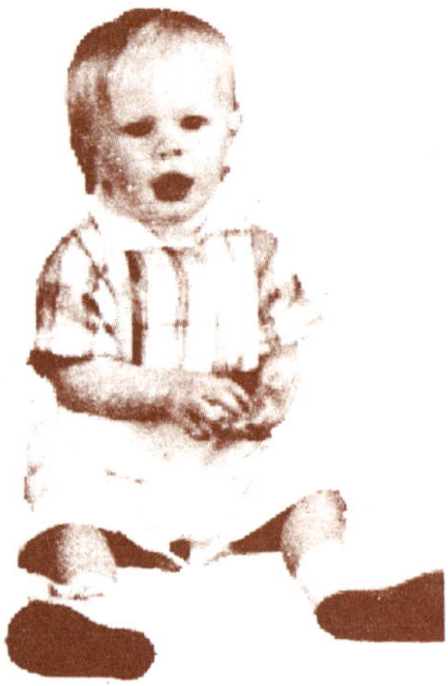

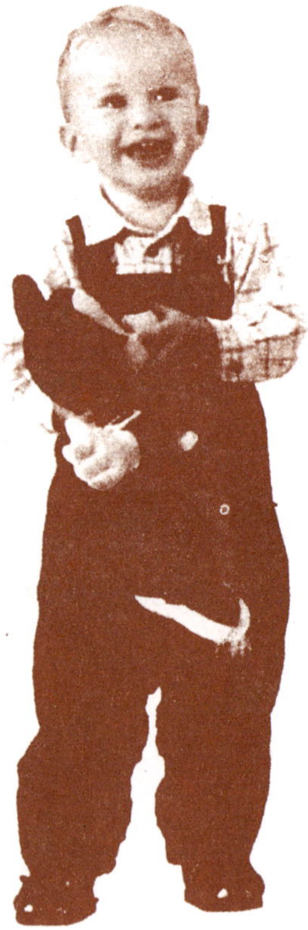

1

Principles of Ayurveda

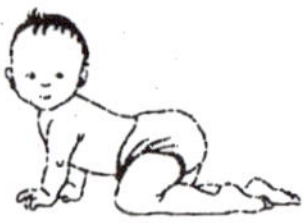

1) Introduction

Ayurveda, is composed of two words viz. Ayu and Veda. Ayu means life and Veda denotes to the science.

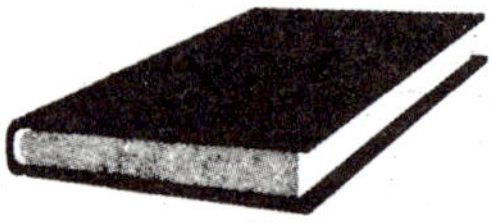

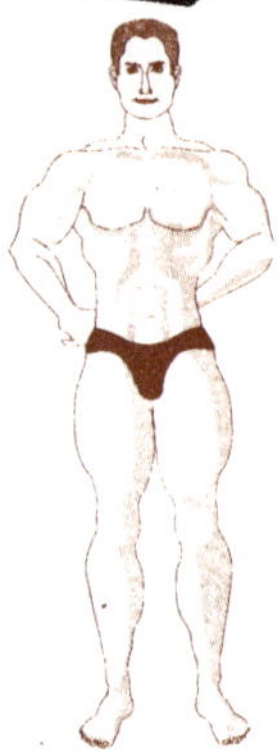

Ayu is defined as a combination of Sharira (body), Indriya (senses), Satva (mind) and Atma (Soul) (spirit). Body without senses, mind and spirit is dead and it is not Ayu.

Ayurveda has mainly three aims viz. first to preserve the health, second to promote the health of the healthy persons and third to cure the disease of the patient. It fulfils these aims through 8 Branches viz. Kayachikitsa (medicine), Shalya Tantra (surgery), Shalakya Tantra (otorhinolaryngology and ophthalmology), Kaumara Bhritya (paediatric and obstetric), Rasayanas (Rejuvination), Vajikarana (revitalisation), Agada Tantra (toxicology) and Bhuta Vidya (Psychology). Out of these generally Rasayana and Vijikarana including Svasthavrutta deal with the preservation and promotion of the health of the healthy persons and the remaining branches deal with the diseased person.

2) Pancha Mahabhuta

From the Indian philosophical point of view all the matters of the universe are made up of 5 elements, collectively

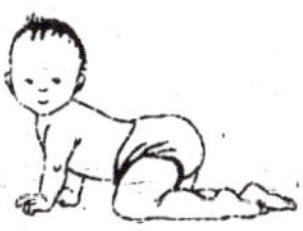

known as Pancha Mahabhuta (five basic elements). These are Akasha, Vayu, Tejas, Jala and Pruthvi. Each of these can be perceived by its distinctive quality viz. Akasha by Shabda (sound), Vayu by Sparsha (touch), Agni by Roopa (form as seen) Jala by Rasa (taste) and Pruthvi by Gandha (odour) (Aroma).

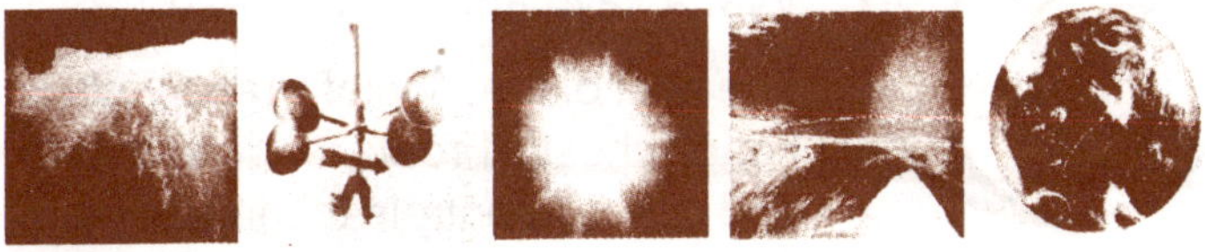

3) Dosha

The concept of Dosha has been evolved by the great sages of Ayurveda to differentiate with living and not-livings. Though Sharira (human body) is made of Pancha Mahabhuta, It attains life only when Atma (spirit) (Soul), Indriya (senses) and Mana (mind) joint it. Dosha are the biological units of the living body which are responsible for its all functions. Dosha are three viz. Vata, Pitta and Kapha and each of which is also made up of Mahabhuta. Vayu and Akasha Mahabhuta form Vata. Agni Mahabhuta form Pitta and Pruthvi and Jala Mahabhuta form Kapha Dosha.

The word Dosha is derived from the verb 'Dusa' which means to vitiate. In the normal state of equilibrium they support the body and when vitiated produce the disease. Dosha play important role in the pathogenesis, diagnosis and treatment of the diseases.

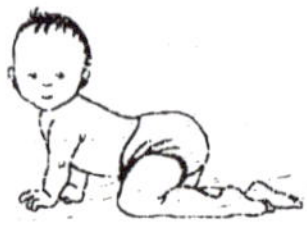

Vata

The word 'Vata' is derived from the verb 'Va' which means Gati (motion). This Dosha is responsible for all the movements in the body. It is of 5 types viz. Prana Vayu, Udana Vayu, Samana Vayu, Vyana Vayu and Apana VAyu.

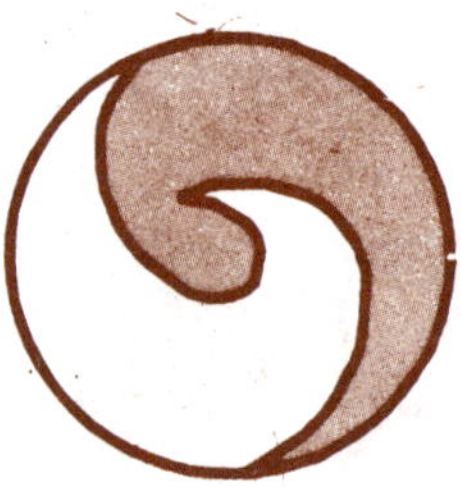

The seat of function of Prana Vayu is head, chest, throat, tongue, mouth and nose. It controls the functions of salivation, eructation, sneezing, respiration, deglutition etc. The seat of function of Udana Vayu is umbilicus, chest and throat. Its main function is phonation. It also provides enthusiasm, vitality, complexion etc. to the human beings.

Functions of Samana Vayu are closely related to Agni (digestive-juices). It regulates the secretion of the gastric juice, retains the food in the stomach or intestine for the required time, thus helps in its absorption. Vyana Vayu which is situated all over the body is responsible for pulsation of heart and blood circulation. It also controls the movement of eyes, limbs etc.

The seat of function of Apana Vayu are testes, urinary bladder, umbilical region, thigh, groin etc. It controls the functions of elimination of the semen, urine, faeces etc. The movements related with the delivery of foetus are also governed by it.

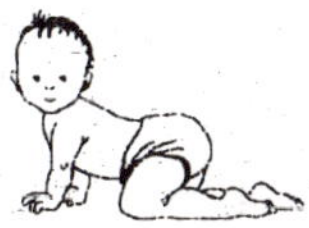

Pitta

The word 'Pitta' is derived from the root 'Tapa' which means heat (Santapa). This Dosha is responsible for digestion and metabolism of the body. It is of 5 types viz. Pachaka Pitta, Ranjaka Pitta, Bhrajaka Pitta, Alochaka Pitta and Sadhaka Pitta.

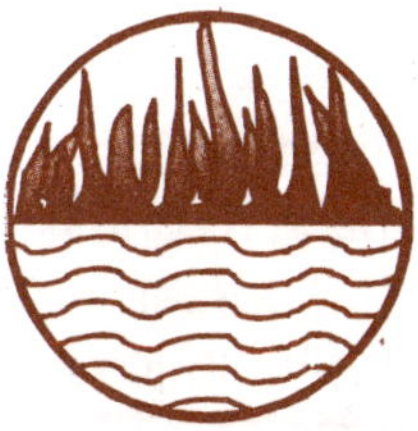

Pachaka Pitta is located in the Grahani (stomach and intestine). Its main function is digestion and is also augments the other Pitta situated in the body. Seats of function of Ranjaka Pitta are liver and spleen. Its main function is to convert Rasa into Rakta (blood). Bhrajaka Pitta is found in the skin and it provides pigmentation to the skin, hair etc.

Alochaka Pitta is situated in the eye, and vision and discrimination of colours are its functions. Sadhaka Pitta is located in the Hridaya and it is responsible for intelligence and ego. It is due to this Pitta that all the functions of the mind and body are co-ordinated.

Kapha

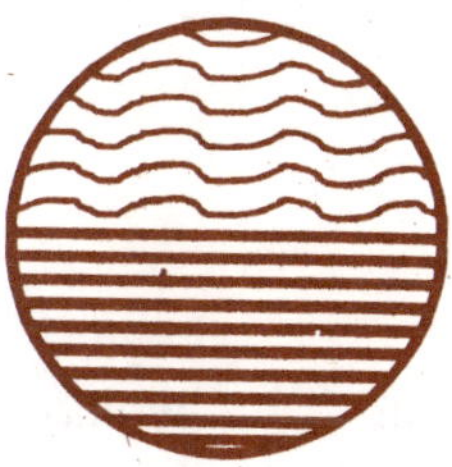

Kapha is also called Shleshma. One of its main functions is to provide nutrition to the bodily tissues. Kapha is also of five types viz. Kledaka Kapha, Avalambaka Kapha, Tarpaka Kapha, Bodhaka Kapha and Shleshaka Kapha.

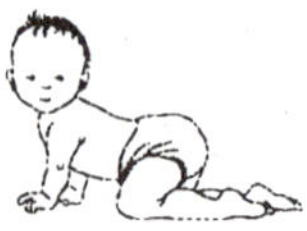

Kledaka Kapha is situated in the stomach. It is slimy (Picchila) in quality, sweet in taste and has the action of moistening the food ingested. It also protects the digestive organs from being hurt by the digestive juices.

Avalambaka Kapha is located in the chest where it provides the norishment to the heart. Bodhaka Kapha is found in the tongue and it is responsible for perceiving the taste. Seat of function of Shleshaka Kapha in joints where it lubricates the joints so that they may function properly. Tarpaka Kapha is situated in the head and gives nutrition to the mental faculties.

Manas Dosha

In addition to Vata, Pitta and Kapha which are the bodily Dosha, there are two Manas Dosha viz. Rajas (passion) and Tamas (darkness). Manas Dosha may be held responsible for mental diseases.

4) Dhatu

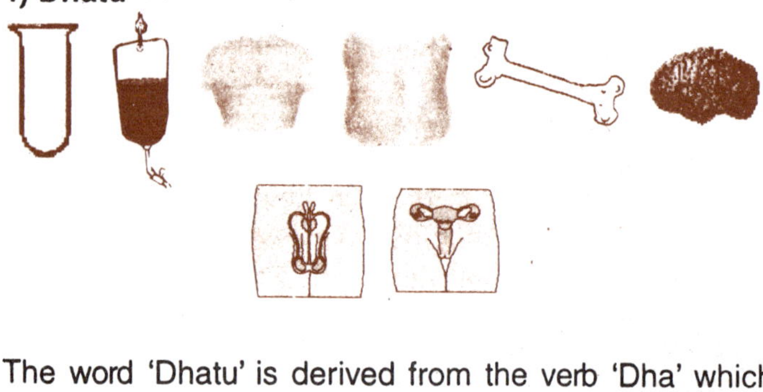

The word 'Dhatu' is derived from the verb 'Dha' which means to hold. The matters which hold the body are termed as Dhatu. In general, it is a term signifying bodily

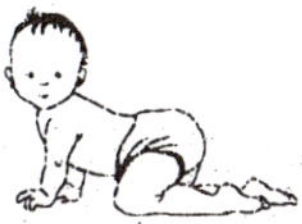

fluids and tissues. Dhatu are of seven types viz. Rasa (nourishing fluid of plasma), Rakta (blood), Mamsa (muscular tissue), Meda (fatty tissue), Asthi (bone and connective tissues), Majja (bone marrow) and Shukra (vital substance/reproductive tissue).

There are three types of pathological changes in these Dhatu viz. Kshaya (decrease), Vruddhi (increase) and Prakopa (Vitiation). The Kshaya of the one and Vruddhi of other may be simultaneous in the same disease and in the same patient. In this condition, the Dhatu increases at one place at the cost of other.

5) Upadhatu

Upadhatu are actually not nourishing the body but they are the by-products of Dhatu, necessary for supporting the body. They are Stanya (breast milk), Artava (menstrual blood), Kandara (tendons), Sira (vessels), Vasa (fat), Twak (skin), Snayu etc. They are also vitiated by Dosha.

6) Mala

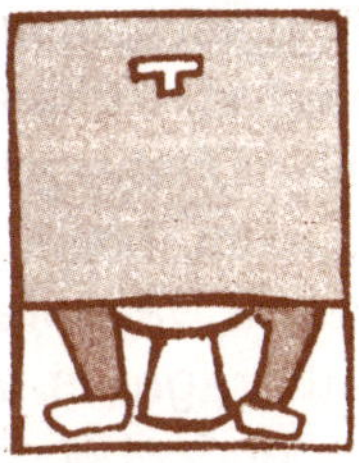

Mala are different exccretions viz. faeces, urine, Mala Kapha, Mala Pitta, excretions from organs, Sweda (sweat), Nakha (nails), hair, the oily discharge from skin etc. The Mala are also get vitiated and included in Dushya.

7) Srotas

The word 'Srota' is derived from 'Sru'

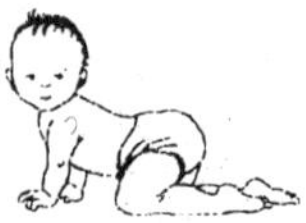

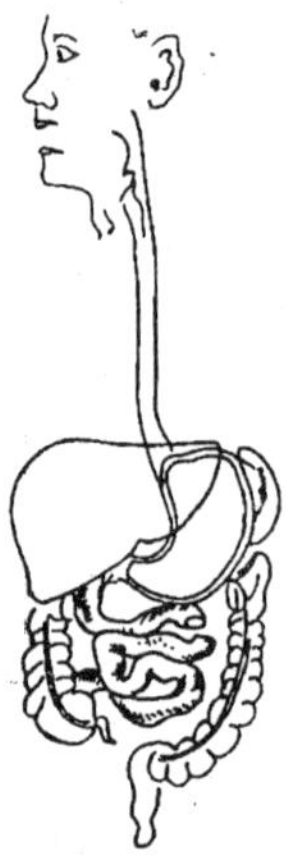

which means oozing. The oozing of nourishing fluid and the return of waste matters take place through these Srotas. In fact, the whole body is composed of Srotas, but for the convenience of diagnosis and treatment, they have been classified in 13 groups. They are Prana-Vaha (channels through which oxygen and carbon dioxide exchange take place), Udaka-Vaha (water-balance), Anna-Vaha (food passage), Rasa-Vaha, Rakta-Vaha, Mamsa-Vaha, Meda-Vaha, Asthi-Vaha, Majja-Vaha, Shukra-Vaha, Mutra-Vaha (urinary channels), Purisha-Vaha (channel for faeces) and Sweda-Vaha (channels for sweat).

8) Agni

Agni is a very important factor because Ayurveda believes that majority, if not all the diseases are caused by disturbance of Agni. It is responsible for all the digestion and metabolism of the body. It is of 13 types viz. Jatharagni (digestive juices), Seven Dhatvagni i. e. Agni of Rasa, Rakta, Mamsa, Meda, Asthi, Majja and Shukra and 5 Bhutagni i. e. Agni of Akasha, Vayu, Tejas, Jala and Pruthvi. Out of these, Jatharagni is very important and all the other Agni are dependant upon it.

The vitiation of these Agni are of three types viz. Vishamagni, Tikshnagni and Mandagni. These three

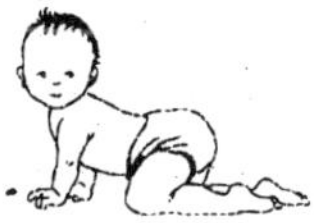

abnormalities of Agni are responsible for producing the various types of diseases but Mandagni is the common cause of most of the diseases.

9) Aama

Aama has been defined (i) undigested or half/semi-digested food (ii) Mala-Sanchaya (the accumulation of excretory products) and (iii) first vitiation of Dosha. Generally, it is produced by diminished power of digestive juices (Mandagni), but it may also from at other levels of the Agni i.e. Bhutagni and Dhatvagni.

In short, Aama may be produced at any level of digestion and metabolism. It is also a frequent cause of the diseases. Great stress has been laid in Ayurveda on correction of the digestion. The word Kaya-Chikitsa means treatment of vitiated Agni as Kaya means Jatharagni and Chikitsa means treatment.

(16)

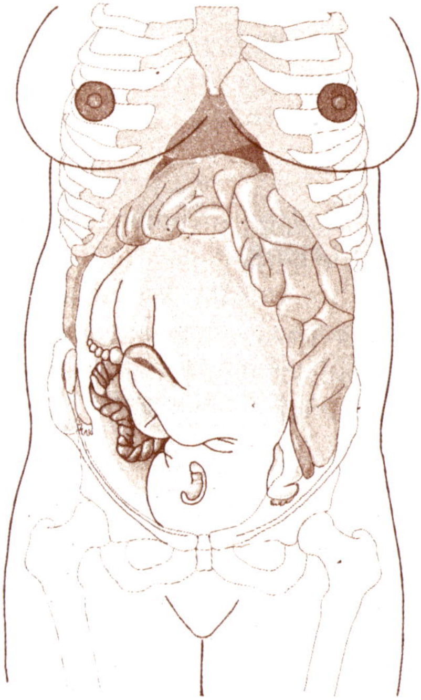

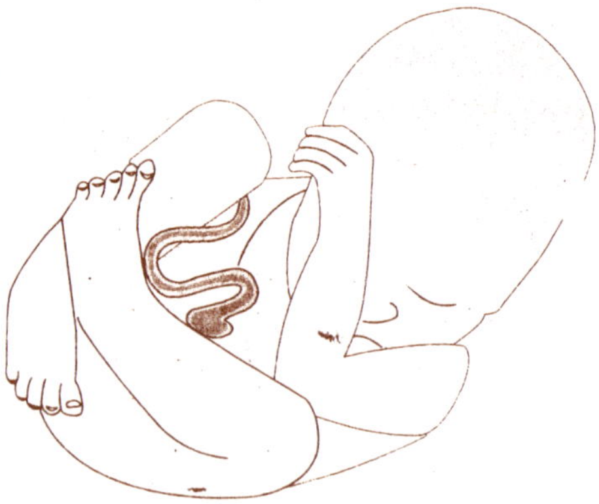

2

Embryology (Garbha-Hetu Vijnana)

(discussion on the causation of the foetus)

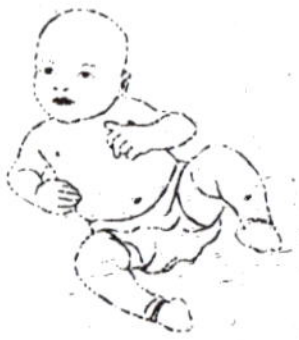

1) Assemblage of materials required for the creation of the foetus

The creation of the foetus is assured if the following four essentials are present and combine in a proper manner. (1) the genetic period (Ritu) (2) the uterus (3) normal female secretion (ovum) and (4) the male seed.

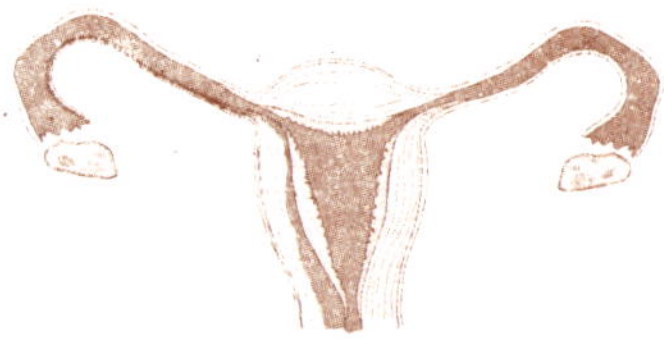

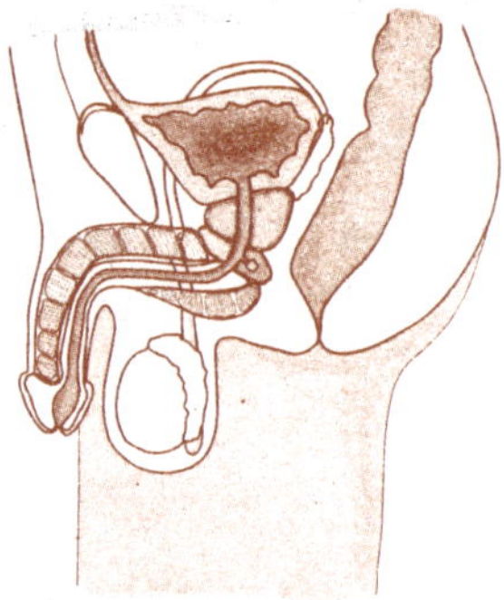

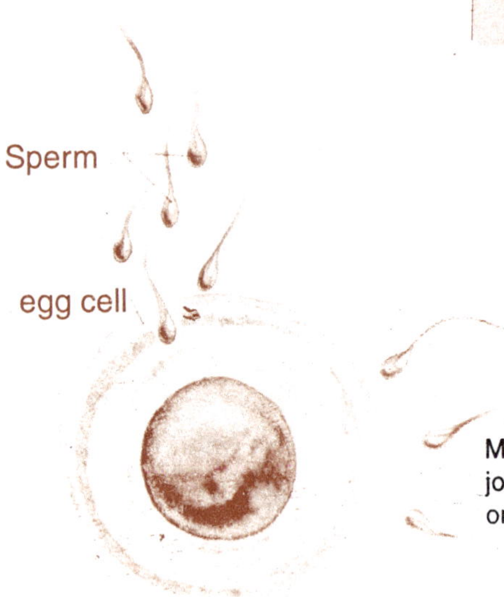

Many **sperm cells** try to join with the **egg cell,** but only one will get in.

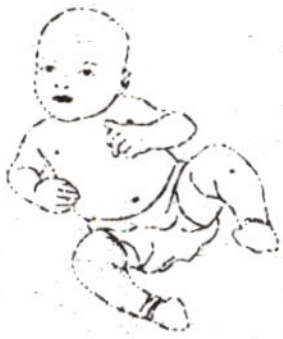

The growth of the foetus resembles that of the sprout which shoots out if (1) a good seed is sown (2) in a moist soil and (3) at the proper season. The woman acts like a field (kshetra) and the man like a seed which is sown. The creation of all beings is due to the proper union of the seed and the field.

(S. Sa. 2 & Ms. 9)

Ritu (genetic period) means a state of the female body which indicates the proper time for conception, menstruation is its outward manifestation. A woman here called Kshetra is really the best aphrodisiac and stimulant for procreation.

(C. Ci. 2)

The human seed is a conglomeration of various minute parts representing the structures of the body. The being that is produced is thus a replica of the parent.

(Chakradatta)

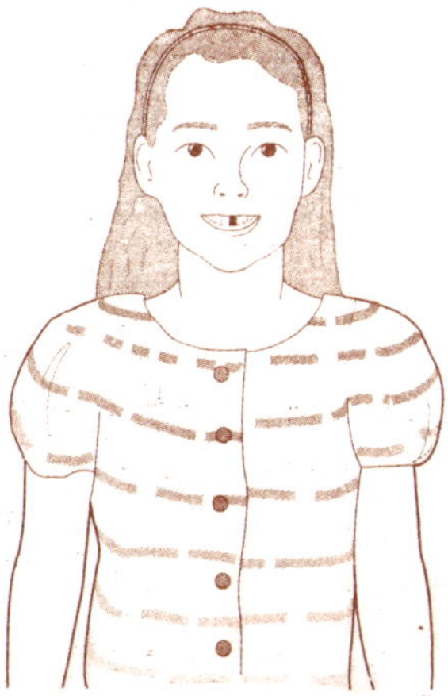

A woman begets a stout son when all essentials viz. the uterus, the path of the ovum, the female and male seed, vata and the mental state are normal and clear.

(A. Hr. Sa. 1)

Ayurveda mentions divisions in the seed, which is noteworthy.

Ritu extends for twelve nights after the first apperance of the

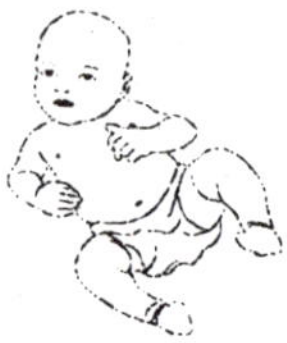

menses, there may not however, in some cases, be any flow of menses.

(S. Sa. 3)

Just as at the end of the day, the lotus always closes its petals, the female passage (yoni) closes itself slightly.

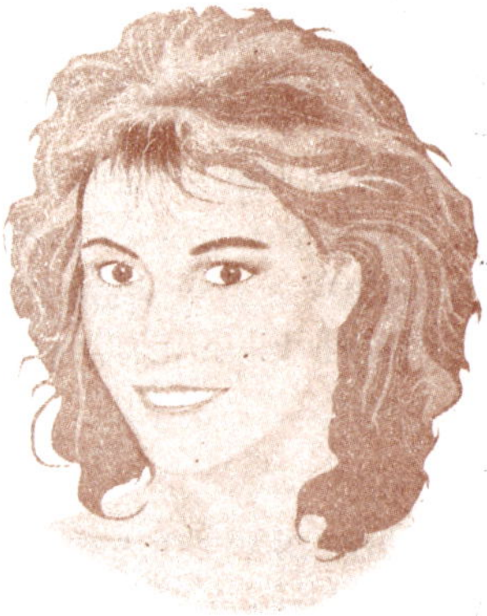

The menses according to Ayurveda keep on generating for a month and accumulate; they are darkish, have a peculiar smell and are conveyed by channels (dhamani) to the mouth of the vagina (yoni). They are produced from fluids of the body (rasa) and flow out for three days in every lunar month.

It appears in young girls at the age of twelve and ceases at the age of fifty, on account of decay of old age.

(S. Sa. 3)

A woman with ritu 'on', can be known by peculiar signs and symptoms.

2) The mental characteristics of the woman who conceives

i) The child resembles the first man she sees on the 4th day of menstruation. She should therefore look at her husband before she begins the day.

(S. Sa. 2)

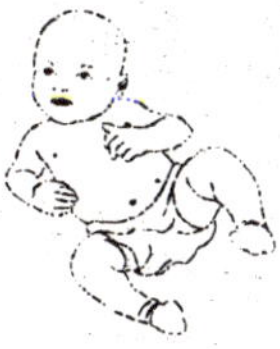

ii) A woman should have a clear picture before her mind of the future child she is going to give birth to; keep her mind engaged on it; should behave according to her ideal of the future child; should hear the description of such a child often enough.

(C. Sa. 8)

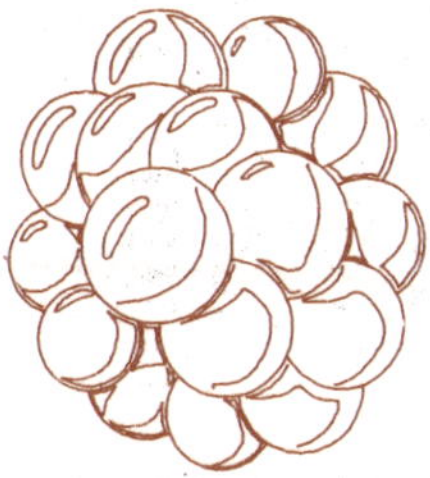

3) The effect of diet on the foetus

The child born to a couple partakes of their habits, behaviour, activities and food tendencies.

(S. Sa. 2)

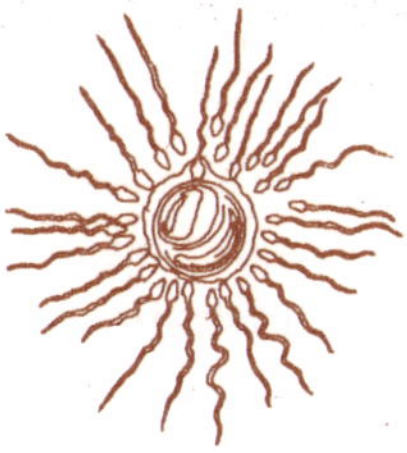

4) Recollection of previous birth

The theory of re-birth : Those who in their former life were always honestly imbued with truth and learning, are born with noble instincts and retain a memory of previous births. A person gets in this life what in his former life he had deserved by his acts. He also acquires those qualities which he had striven for, or to which he was accustomed.

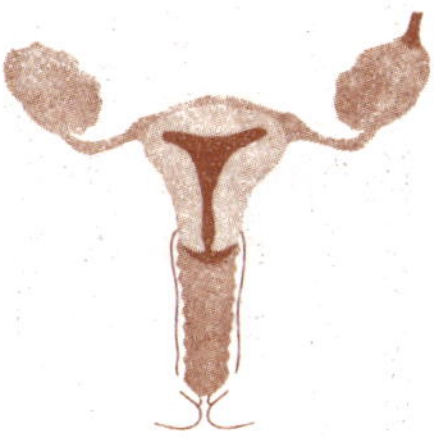

(S. Sa. 2)

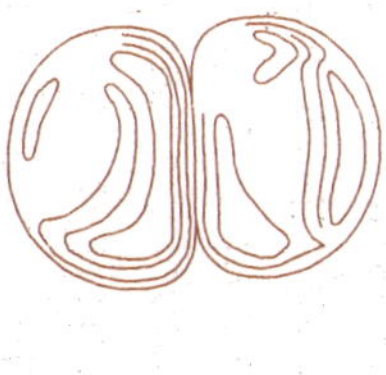

The jiva passes after death from one body to another with hundreds of times, desires and hopes, just like birds who fly from one tree to another.

(Y. V.)

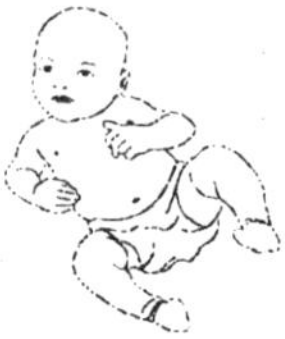

5) Proper age for procreation

The seeds in man and woman mature at the age of 25 and 16 respectively. A physician should know this well. If parents are below this age, the foetus does not develop, dies early or becomes deformed.

(S. Sa. 35)

6) Purity of seeds and of organs

A healthy foetus is formed by union with a man of powerful seed by a woman with uninfected vagina, uterus and menses (ovum).

(C. Sa. 3)

7) The qualities of Shukra and Artava

Shukra (semen) has the quality of being white like Soma and Artava is red like fire. All elements are also present in them inminute degrees. These elements have the natural attribute of helping and strengthening each other and intermingling with them.

(S. Sa. 3)

The presence of the female seed (Artava) in the formation of Garbha - Just as a ball of ghee melts when placed near a fire, similarly the female seed is set forth in coition with man.

(S. Sa. 3)

8) Garbhavakranti

Creation of the foetus : Vayu releases during copulation the Tejas energy of the body and this uniting with vayu,

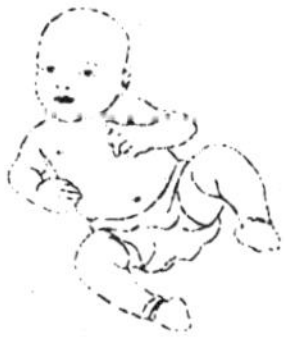

ejects semen. This enters the female passage and combines with Artava. The embryo which develops from this, is thus a combination of Soma and Agni and lodges in the uterus.

(S. Sa. 3)

It is only when Jiva (life) descends in this combination of Shukra and Artava, that a foetus begins to form.

(C. Sa. 3)

Jiva is called (1) Khsetrajna because it resides in the body (Kshetra). It is called (2) a Sentient (power of feeling). Being, as it perceives objects by the senses of touch, smell, sight, sound and taste. (3) It is also the producer, the mover, the seer, substainer or the speaker. Whatever the name, it is eternal, incomprehensible and imperishable.

Owing to its predestined union with the gross elements and the three qualities - Sattva, Rajas and Tamas, it becomes endowed with a character (1) wholly divine or partly so; or (2) demoniac and impelled by vayu, enters the uterus and stays there.

(S. Sa. 3)

9) Theories about a Male or Female issue

During procreation when semen (Shukra) exceeds the female fluid (Artava) in energy, the issue is male; it is a female, when artava is more powerful. The issue is impotent when both energies are equally balanced.

(S. Sa. 3)

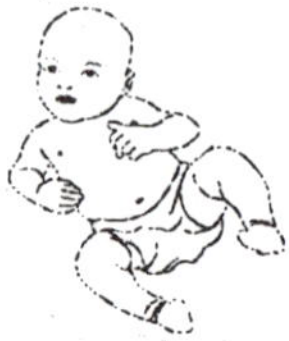

10) What is Garbha (Foetus)

It is the coalescence of the male and female seeds in the uterus where the soul combines with them intimately alongwith the eight Prakrutis (elementary principles) sixteen formations of Prakruti (Vikaras). The eight prakrutis are Avyakta, Mahat, Ahankara and five Tanmatras. The sixteen Vikaras are the five Mahabhutas and the eleven Indriyas.

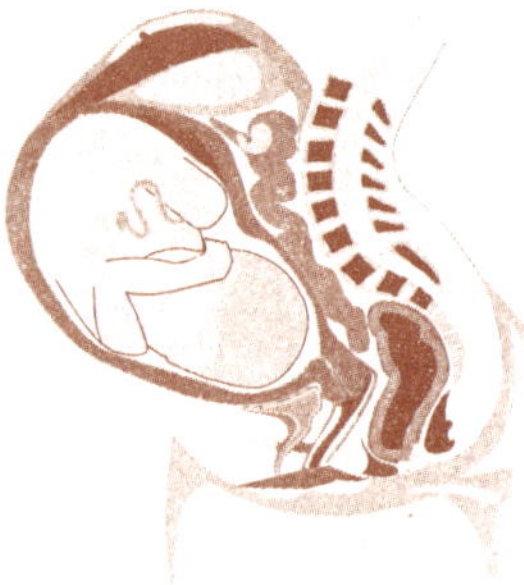

(S. Sa. 5)

11) The functions of the five Mahabhutas in the development of the Foetus

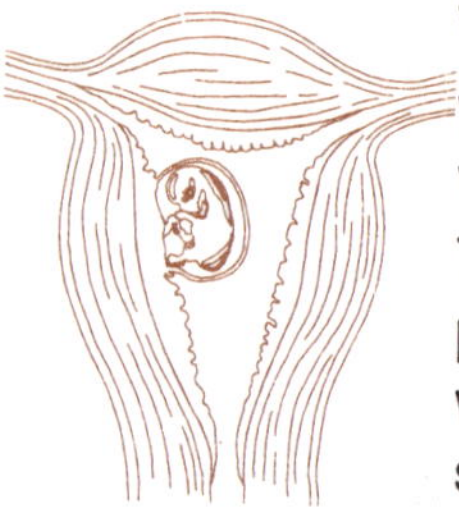

When Garbha is actively energetic, Vayu forms further segmentation. Tejas performs the digestive processes, Apa (water) moisten the whole, the earthy principle (Prithivi) strengthens it and Akasha (space) develops the same.

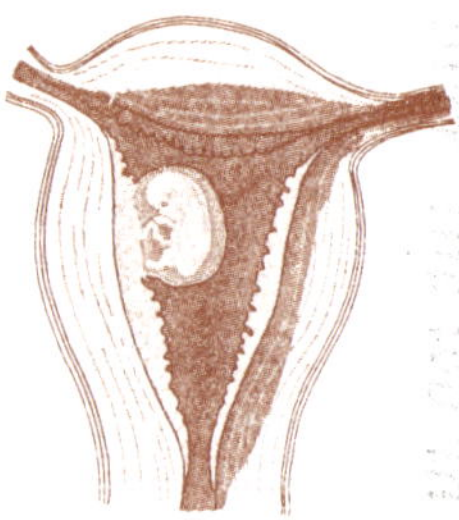

The embryo is styled a body (Sharira) only when it is thus developed with hands, feet, tongue, nose, ears, buttocks and other organs.

(S. Sa. 5)

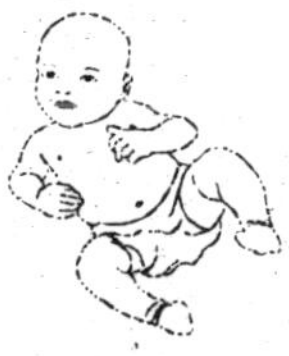

12) The method of formation of Twins or Multiple progeny

When Vayu divides the seed itself in two, a 'twin' results. Both lack proper development. In this process of segmentation, the number of children born is according to the number of divisions in the primitive Garbha (Shukrartava).

(S. Sa. & A. Sm. Sa. 2)

KALALA is the formless mass; when Vayu becomes powerful and divides the mass in two, a twin results (Kris-Atreya).

(Bhel.)

13) The nature of complexion of Garbha

Tejo-Dhatu is the cause of the nature of complexion and is determined at the time of co-habitation; the complexion is fair, if this is watery. It is dark, when Tejas assumes an earthy form. It is shady when this is earthy and partakes of Akasha (space). When Aap (water) and Akasha (space) are prominent, it is fair and dark. According to some, the colour of the food of the pregnant woman determines the colour of the child.

The colour of the eyes also differs according the influence of Tejas. If this enters the sight (drushti) region, blindness results. If it enters Rakta, the eyes are blood-red, tawny (brownish yellow), if mixed with Pitta (bile), white if mixed with Kapha, and awry if Vayu enters the same.

(S. Sa. 2)

Differences in colour of the complexion vary according

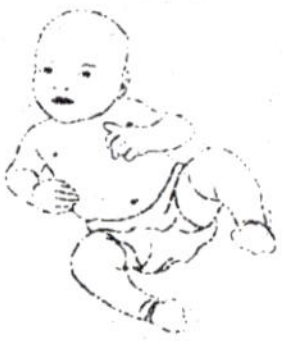

to the influence of the country, the time and the behaviour of the couple.

14) Early signs of Pregnancy

Exhaustion, languor (weakness), thirst, feeling of weakness in thighs and throbbing sensation in the genetic passage.

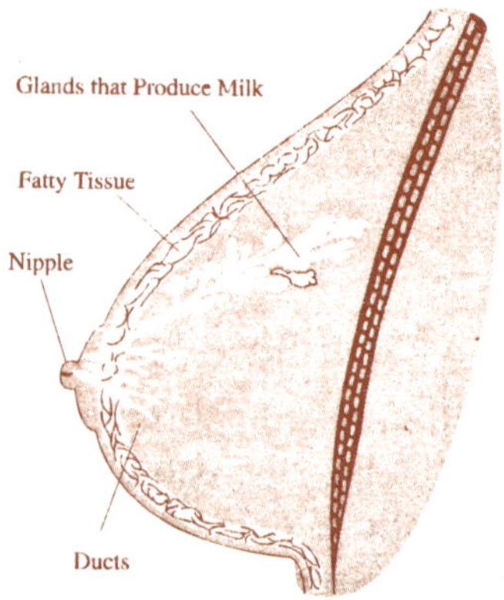

15) Signs and Symptoms in advanced Pregnancy

The signs are : (i) The nipples of the breasts become dark in colour (ii) Breasts develop and grow larger in size and have a milky secretion (iii) The hair stand out on the body (iv) The eye-lids droop (v) 'Quickening' - a feeling of movement in the uterus, occurs from the fourth month onwards. There is itching or burning sensation, due to Dosas formed by the presence of Garbha reaching the heart of the mother; Striae Gravidarum (kikvisa) are also due to the same cause.

The Symptoms are : (i) Voimiting without a cause (ii) A dislike for fragrance (iii) Waterning of the mouth and (iv) Lassitude; menstruation also stops.

(S. Sa. 3; A. Sm. Sa. 4; A. Hr. Sa. 1)

16) Absence of Menstruation and Formation of Placenta

When a woman conceives, the Garbha blocks the outlets

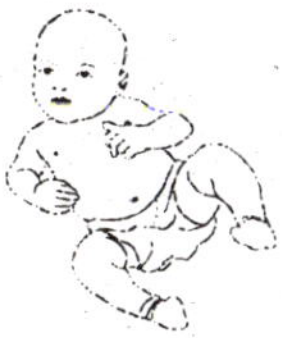

of srotasas of the Artava (menses) and menstruation disappears. When thus obstructed in the lower part, it accumulates, comes tothe upper part of the uterus and forms the placenta (apara). The rest of the Artava rises still upwards in the body and causes the breasts to enlarge, which thus become full and prominent.

(S. Sa. 4)

17) Hygiene of Pregnancy

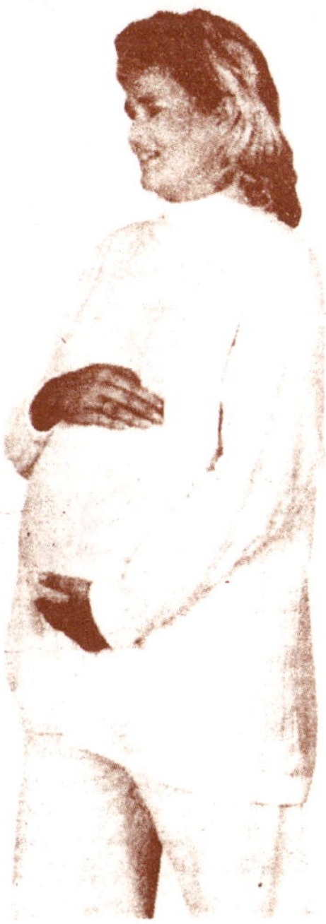

The mother is the chief factor in the development ofthe foetus, which gets all that is good and evil in the mother from conception to delivery.

(Chakra)

If a limb or organ of the mother gets deranged on account of excitment of the Dosas, the same derangement occurs in this foetus.

(S. Sa. 2)

A woman desiring therefore to have a good progeny should avoid all causes of derangement of Doshas e. g. food, and adopt modes of behaviour suited to her condition.

(C. Sa. 8)

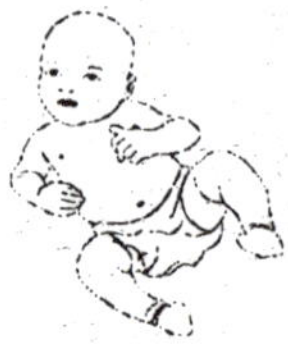

18) Development of Garbha in each month

a) IN THE FIRST MONTH, the embryo is only a "Kalala" (a soft small mass).

b) IN THE SECOND MONTH, the five elements fuse together and by the action of Kapha, Pitta and Vata it becomes more solid.

The mass becomes a compact ball if the child is to be a male. It is moulded like a Pesi, if the child is to be a female. If the child is to be a sexless mass it is irregular in shape.

(S. Sa. 3)

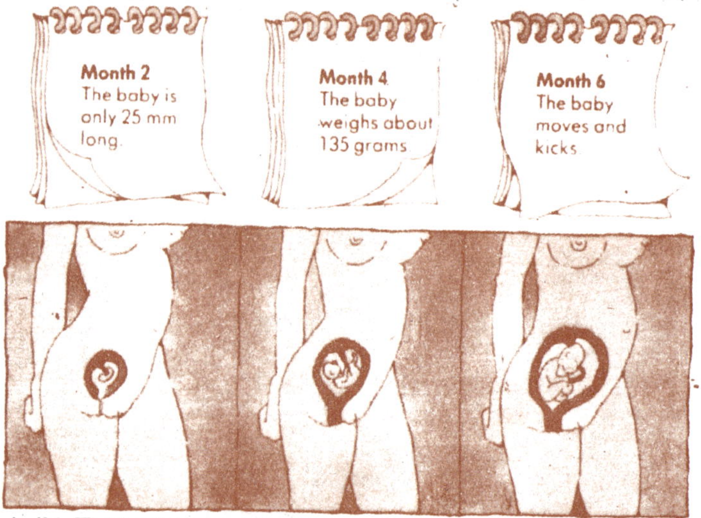

c) IN THE THIRD MONTH, five bud-like protrusions, representing the rudimentary head and limbs, are formed. Other major and subsidiary parts of the body are also indistinctly seen. In this month, also appear all the eleven Indriyas (organs) and all the structures of the body.

(S. Sa. 3; C. Sa. 4)

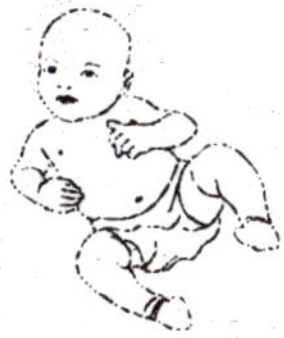

d) IN THE FOURTH MONTH, all organs becomes still more distinct. The heart is now ready to perform all vital functions; the foetus therefore exhibits a desire for various objects, which express themselves as "longings" by the pregnant woman.

e) The pregnant woman has now two hearts; her desires therefore should be satisfied as far as possible; if these desires are fulfilled, the son becomes brave and strong and lives long enough.

The child possesses a body-form and behaviour, similar to the subject, for which the pregnant woman had strong desires or "longings".

(S. Sa. 3)

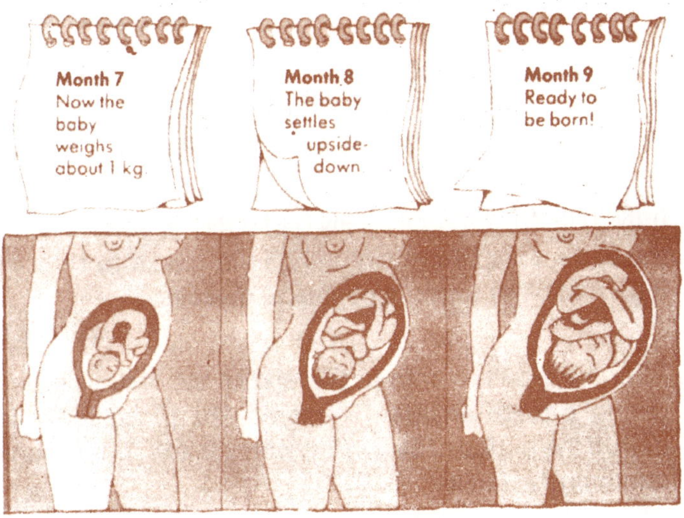

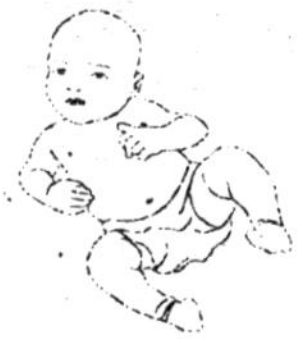

f) IN THE FIFTH MONTH, further development of the powers of the mind takes place; according to Charaka, only the fleshy and muscular parts grow.

(S. Sa. 3; C. Sa. 4)

g) IN THE SIXTH MONTH, according to Shusruta, feelings i. e. powers of perceiving and distinguishing pain and pleasure are evident.

(S. Sa. 3)

Charaka says that accumulation of strength occurs, and complexion to the skin is now imparted.

(C. Sa. 4)

h) IN THE SEVENTH MONTH, further development occurs in the primary and secondary organs. The foetus is now endowed with complete physical structures.

(S. Sa. 3; A. Hr. Sa. 1)

i) IN THE EIGHTH MONTH, Ojas which begins to take a firm hold of the body is itself still unstable. The child if born now, dies, because of want of Ojas.

(S. Sa. 3)

j) IN THE NINETH OR TENTH MONTH, sometimes in the eleventh or twelveth month, a live child may be born; if born at other times, it contracts diseases.

(S. Sa. 3)

After the eighth month to the end of the tenth, delivery can take place any day. These are the proper days for birth. If the period of stay in the womb is exceeded, some abnormality results.

(C. Sa. 4)

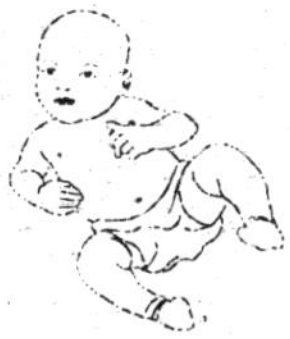

19) Excretion, Respiration and Crying in Intra-uterine life

The excreta are very little in the foetus and Vayu finds no entrance to its colon. It does not therefore defecate, nor urinate, nor pass wind when in the womb.

The mouth of the foetus is covered by Jarayu, the throat by mucus and the passages of Vayu are thus closed. The child does not breathe nor cry in foetal life.

The acts of respiration, movement and sleep are performed by the foetus through similar acts of the mother herself.

(S. Sa. 2)

20) Natural position of the foetus in the uterus

It lies in the uterus with all its body parts bent, the head directed downwards and the face to the back of the mother. At delivery, therefore, it naturally descends head-foremost. This position enables it to occupy the smallest space in the uterus.

(S. Sa. 5; C. Sa. 6)

21) Nutrition of the foetus in the uterus

The cord that enters the naval of the foetus is called the Umbilical Cord. This cord is attached at the other end to the vessels, that contains the essence of nourishing juices derived from mother's food. It is from this nutriment, that the development of the foetus takes place.

Nutrition of the foetus commences from the moment of conception, when even primary and secondary organs

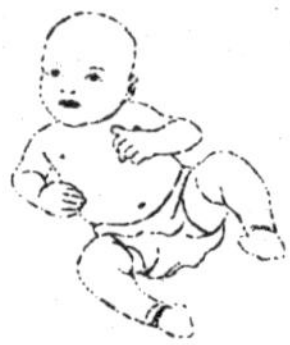

have not appeared. The life-juices are supplied by Rasa-carrying Dhamanis (channels), which go obliquely and are connected with every organ of the body.

(S. Sa. 3)

The cord develops alongwith the primary and secondary organs. It starts from the navel of the foetus and is attached to the placenta, which again is connected indirectly to the heart of the mother. Nourishment thus flows from her heart to the placenta and to the navel of the foetus. It then passes to the Pakvasaya, where it is acted upon by the heart of the foetal body, becomes more vitalised and is enabled to nourish all its own tissues.

(A. Sm. Sa. 2)

The development of the foetus is first due to the above nourishing fluid and secondly to the impetus to vital activity given by Vayu.

Some say that the navel (nabhi) contains the flash of the vital energy; development of the foetus begins when this energy bursts into flame and stimulates every activity.

Vayu combines with Agni (body-heat) and successively separates by fission, the several Srotasas situated in the upper, middle and lower part of the foetus.

(S. Sa. 4)

22) Contributes in the developments of foetus

The parts that contribute in the construction of the foetus are (1) the father (2) the mother (3) the nourishing fluid (4) the vital force (5) the mental faculty (6) the assimilation.

THE FATHER contributes firm parts like the hair, beard,

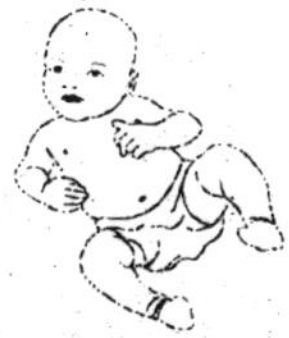

the bones, the nails, the teeth, blood vessels, muscles, dhamani, semen and other similar objects.

THE MOTHER contributes the soft parts viz. flesh, blood, fat, marrow, the brain, heart, navel, liver, spleen, intestines and the anus.

NOURISHMENT produces compactness, strength of body, complexion,sustenance and destruction.

VITALITY produces acuteness of senses, perception, discernment, longevity, power to bear pain and enjoy pleasure.

ASSIMILATION produces vigour, health, strength, colour of the skin and the intellect.

23)The contribution of the five gross elements (Maha-bhutas)

1) Akasha produces sound, sense of hearing and discriminating power.

2) Vata element produces the skin, sense of tough and respiration.

3) Tejas produces sight, perception of colour and form and digestion.

4) Aap produces the tongue, the sense of taste and all secretions in the body.

5) Earth element produces the nose, the sense of smell and bones.

(A. Hr. Sa. 3)

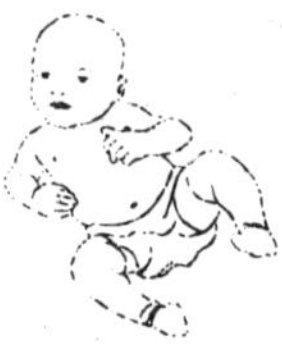

24) Diagnosis of sex of the foetus

The child will be a male when (i) mother gets secretion first in the right breast (ii) has heavyness of right eye (iii) walks with right foot forward (iv) desires articles with a masculine name (v) enjoys and sees lotuses of the best sort (vi) other articles with masculine names and with a pleasing apperance. The child is a female, if the opposite conditions are found.

When the child is neither male or female, the woman shows all signs of pregnancy and also prominence of the abdomen and both sides of the waist.

Diagnosis of Twins

When the middle part of the abdomen sinks inwards like a saucer, twins may be present.

(S. Sa. 3)

Garbha - Vyakaranam
Detailed explanation of the Foetus

1) Pranas and their seats in the body

Pranas (vital elements) are twelve in number (i) agni (or pitta) (ii) sóma (or kapha) (iii) vayu (vata) (iv) satva (v) rajas (vi) tamas (vii) to (xi) the five senses and (xii) the Soul (Bhutatma).

(S. Sa. 4)

Prana is that which imparts life-energy.

Their seats in the body are (i) the head (Murdhan) (ii) the throat (Kantha) (iii) the Heart or Brain (Hridaya) (iv) the

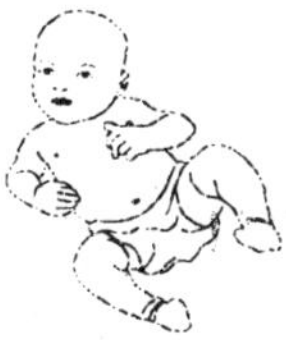

Navel (v) the Anus (Guda) (vi) Urinary Bladder (Basti) (vii) Brightness (Ojas) (viii) the Semen (Shukra) (ix) menstrual fluid (Shonita) (x) flesh (Mamsa). The first six are marmas.

(C. Sa. 7)

CHARAKA in another place mentions two; Sankhas and Rakta instead of the navel, the flesh and the menstrual fluid.

The best physician is one who knows the seats of Pranas, the Indriyas; the knowledge of diseases and their causes, symptoms and treatment and the knowledge of Atman. He can be called Pranabhisar, as he can make the Pranas to return.

(C. Sa. 29)

(36)

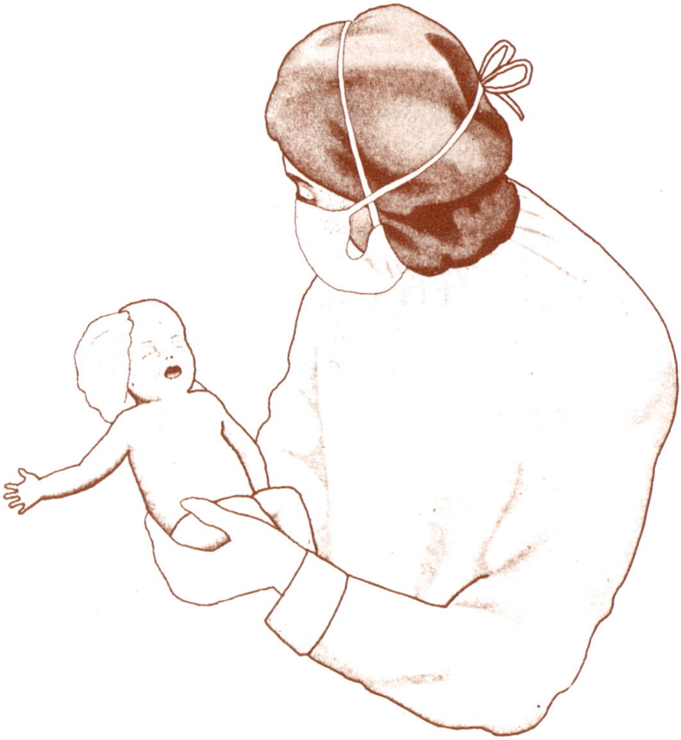

3

New Born Baby care

(Navjat Paricharya)

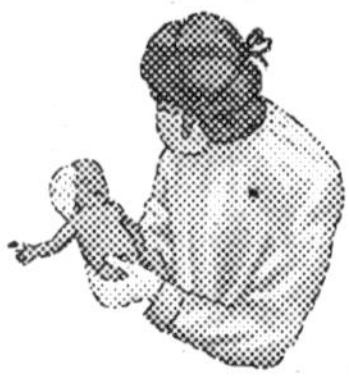

After jatkarm the baby is kept in special room called Kumaragar. The room must be airy, with sufficient light. The baby should be isolated from people. The clothes of baby, even room's clothes must be clean and soft. The baby and room daily fumigated with Vacha (acorus calamus), Ajmoda (carum roxburghianum), Jatamansi (nordiostachys jatamansi) Guggulu (commiphera mukul) called Rakshoghna dhoop. It protects the baby from Devil bodies, Grah-badha, Vranadushti (wound infection).

After jatkarm baby is called Navjat (neonates). During Navjat paricharya attention is given on baby's feeding, Dehoshma (body temperature) prevent it from Sankraman (infection) and observe any signs of illness.

Always keep oleated cotton swab on its frotanell and oil in the ears.

Daily massage with Bala (cida cordifolin) or Chandan bala lakshadi tail. Fine dust powder of Amalaki (emblica officinalis), Haridra (curcuma longa), Kachora (curcuma Zedoaria) mixed in milk apply to the body while bathing. Lukewarm water is used for bath. Fumigation with Ajamoda, Shatpushpa (anethem sowa), Guggulu is done after bath. Fine Vacha powder is applied on its head, back, chest, wrap the baby in soft clean clothes. All these things give baby nice sleep, strength and it can grow properly.

NALKARM (Umbilical cord care)

On nabhi nadi, dusting of fine powder of Haridra, Yashtimadhu (glycyrrhiza-glabra), Ushir (vetiveria

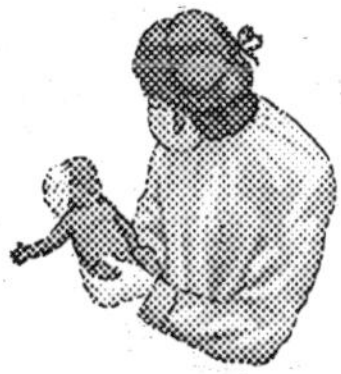

zizanioids) is done and wrapped loosely with clean, soft cloth. If it is wet, after urination or passing stool, change it immediately. Do not allow dust particles or flies to sit on it.

MAL-MUTRA PRAVRUTTI (Defaecation - urination)

First 24 to 48 hours after birth, watch its mal-mutra pravruti. First three days sanchit mal (accumulated waste products) is coming out. Afterwards mal excreted is from baby's own aahar (food), it's nature is different, colour converts from blackish to yellowish.

AAHAR (Diet)

According to agnibal (digestive power) aahar should be given. Stanya pravruti (Breast milk) is after 3 days. First 3 days baby feeds with navnit (butter), First day baby's handful of butter medicated with Laxmana (   ) drug should be given thrice a day alongwith honey. Second day, same quantity of butter medicated with ananta (   ) alongwith honey is given. Third day stanya pravartan takes place. First stanya, called piyush which is heavy (not easily digested), picchil (sticky), ghan (thick), abhishyandi (moisture producing) and less fat quantity, so baby might get loose motion. That is why, though stanya pravartan is there, navnit should be given twice a day, it controlls the loose motion. Laxmana and ananta are nourishing and protect the baby from grahbandha.

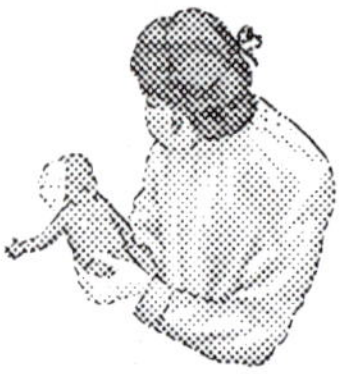

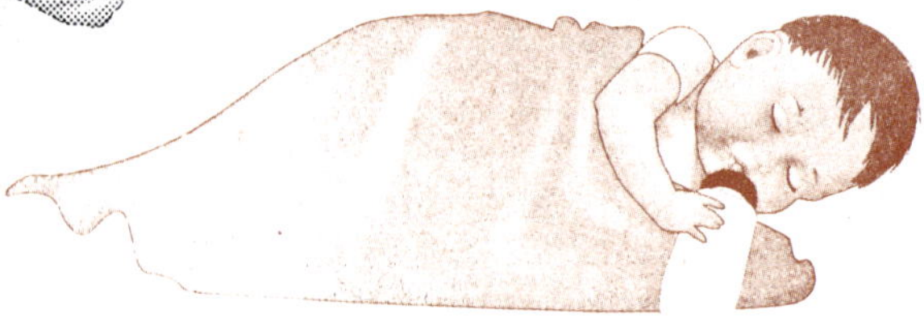

MEDICINE

- Boiled water with gold and give it to baby.
- Ingredients of Balguti (mixture of plants) rubbed in milk or water and give it to baby.
- Powder of Gold, Shankhpushpi (convolvulus pluricaulis), Vacha (acorus calamus), Ashwagandha (withonia somnifera), Jatamansi (nordiostachys jatamansi) should be given with honey and Ghrut once a day. It is useful for baby's health, strength, intelligence and memory.

4

Health care of Child (Prenatal, Postnatal and Food)

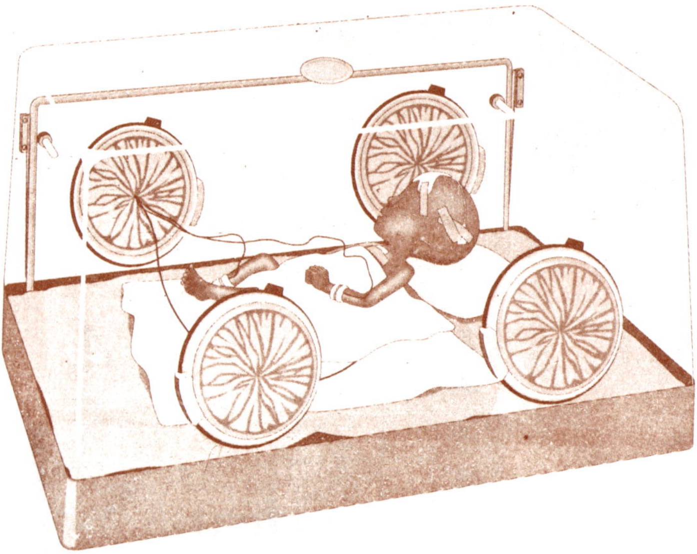

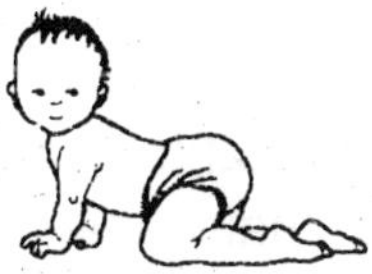

1) Kumaragar - Baby room

i) Spacious House.

ii) Clean (Sterile).

iii) Equiped with useful instruments.

iv) Quiet Place.

v) Good ventilation.

vi) Experienced old woman.

vii) Lady doctor.

viii) Washed & purified/sterile, dried and soft clothes.

ix) Bed clothes/coverings - Fumigated - Sterile with medicated smoke.

(A. S. U. A. - 1)

2) Diet of Child

i) First Day - Honey + Ghee ... three times a day. Mix Anant plant powder (a pinch) in it chant Mantras (positive approach) and give to the child for licking.

(A. U. I.)

ii) Second day - Give above mixture mixed with Laxmana plant.

iii) Third day - Ghee be given. Breast milk followed by butter.

(A. U. I. 1 - 13.14)

3) Mother's Milk (Breast Milk)

Breast milk of mother is advised. It is useful for body growth.

(V. U. 1.13)

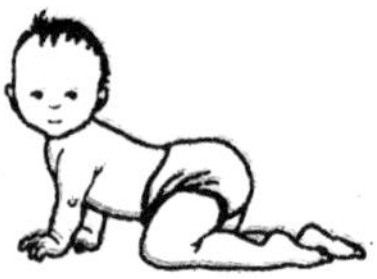

4) Milk

i) Milk of animals is assimilable and good as it is from living animals (animal kingdom).

ii) Milk is

a) Disease remover/corrector.

b) Provides strength - anabolic.

c) Aphrodisiac - Vajikara.

d) Rasayana - Rejuvinator.

e) Improve Intelligence.

(S. S. 35-29)

5) Child - Time Slot

Three times

i) Kshreerapa - Fed on only milk - 1 st year.

ii) Ksheerannada - Fed on milk & food - 2nd year.

iii) Annada - Mainly on Food - 3rd year onwards.

(S. S. 35-29)

6) i) Mother with no Breast milk.

ii) Mother with less Breast milk.

iii) Vitiated milk of mother.

iv) Difficult child birth with debility. hence

v) Suffering from some disease.

To get Breast milk to the child

Use of DHATRI (WET NURSE), young, loving to children, of good health, delivered a child nearly the same time, having sufficient milk for child.

(A. S. U. I.)

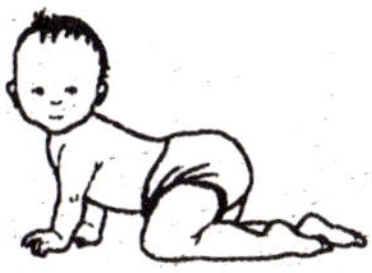

7) Withdrawal of Breast milk

Ataining age of 10 months gradually withdraw Feeding breast milk and replace gradually Light (Laghu) & nutritious (Brimhan) food with milk be started.

(A. S. U. I.)

8) i) Honey,

ii) Sugar candy and

iii) Priyal (Buchaninia latifolia) mixed together be given to child.

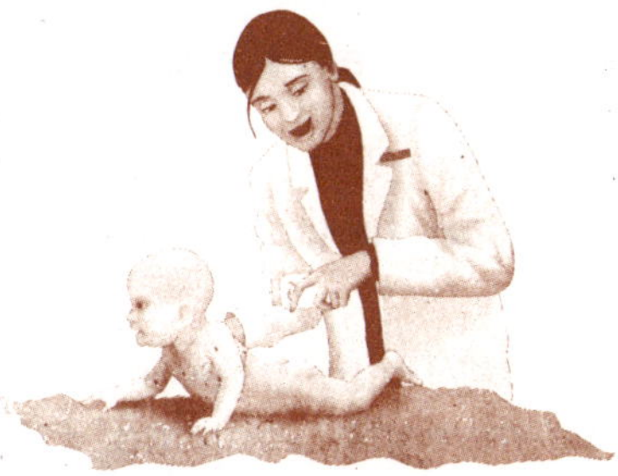

9) Child care taker should be

i) Trained

ii) Good behaved

iii) Not too obese

iv) Not greedy

v) Dutyful

vi) Concentration on child and they are good,

having opposite qualities are bad for child and make the child sick.

(A. S. U. I.)

10) Toys for the child

i) Having sound

ii) Pleasant

iii) Large size

iv) Blunt (Not sharp)

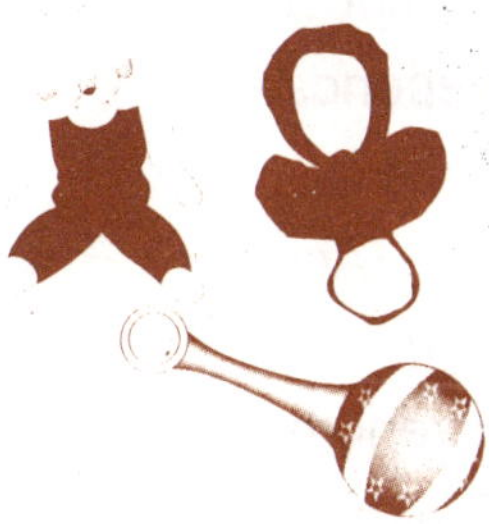

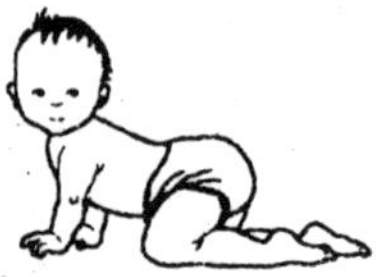

v) Animals

vi) Fruits

vii) Clean (Not dirty)

viii) Uneven, without vaccume

ix) Not hot

x) Not contaminated with wind, rain, dust, smoke and water.

(S. S. 10-47)

11) Teeth

i) Teeth erruption starts in 4th month. Delayed in weak child.

ii) Uneven, too small, too broad teeth are not good.

Ideal teeth

Equal, solid, lustourus, oily, clean, healthy, strong and redish gums.

Time of eruption is disease period/Time i. e. Fever, Thirst, Conjuctivitis, cough, loose motions, vomiting, skin problem like - Eresepalas.

12) Dosage of Medicine in child

A) i) Not specified

ii) Depends on

a) Time

b) Fire (Agni)

c) Age

d) Strength

e) Prakruti

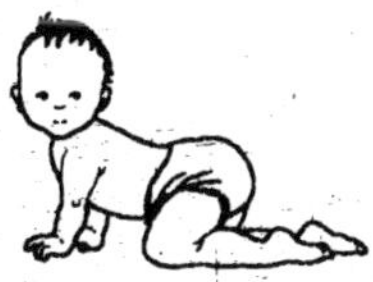

f) Dosha

g) Desh (area)

B) Time to administer medicine

Five types

i) Sunrise (Morning)

ii) Day time meal (Breakfast/Lunch)

iii) Sunset (Evening) (Dinner)

iv) On & off - Every now & then - often

v) Night

C) According to age

i) First month - 5 mgms - 10 mgms. alongwith Avaleh (Jam), milk, honey, sugar & ghee

ii) Increase dose every year.

iii) At sixteenth year - adult dose.

iv) Continue till 70th year.

v) After 70th year decrease every year like child dose.

(S. P. K.)

(48)

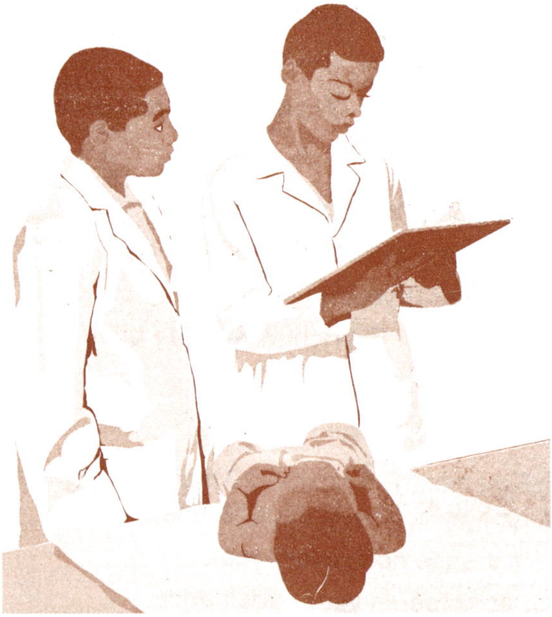

5

Health Tips

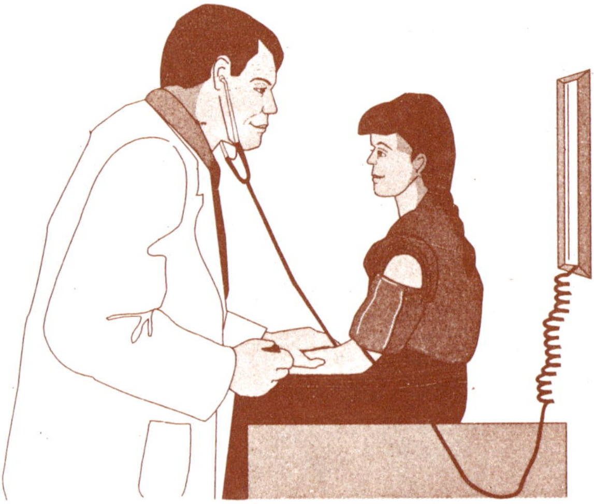

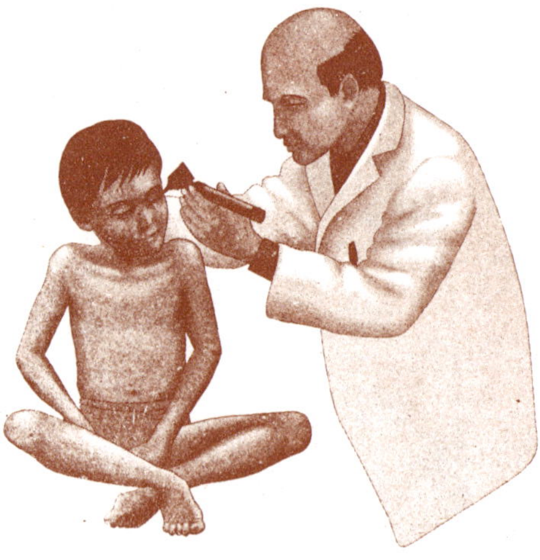

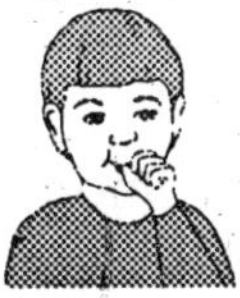

1) Season

Childhood is Kaphkal in human life. (Biological water humor)

Water is formative element, origin of life, responsible for growth, responsible for development.

Excess water produces mucus it indicates poor digestion. Hence diseases of Kapha (Lungs) (Common cold), cough, Bronchitis.

Children may be considered as Kaph Prakruti upto 2 years or 5 years.

2) Diet

Bland/Even

i) Avoid excess of sweet, strong spices overly sour food, too much salt.

ii) Dairy product and sugar

Milk + Spices - good

Cow's

iii) Dairy products - Proteins for vegetarian. Meat can be substituted. Dairy products are mucus forming. Milk, Cheese, Yogurt.

iv) Milk be taken alone.

No good with Bread, sour fruit, beans, nuts, fish and meat.

Good combination with whole grains sweet fruit like bananas.

v) Yogurt does not combine with milk, sour fruit, nuts.

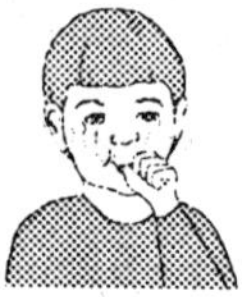

vi) Pasturized milk is like precooked food. More mucus forming as it is devitalised.

Raw milk - boil - spices like Cordmom, cinamon, ginger, cloves is good. A pinch to 1/4 quarter teaspoon + honey or raw sugar is good digestible.

vii) Cold pasturized milk with meal of breads, meats is toxic combination.

vii) Warm milk is good sedative. Add nutmeg 1/4 teaspoon. Milk is mild laxative (Virechan) avoid in conditions of loose motions.

ix) Cheese with cumin, mustard, cyene pepper reduces mocus forming properties.

Cheese is most mucus forming and should not be used in excess.

x) Yogurt - with meals, mixed with fresh cucumbers, Cumin, coriander, cilantro, Cyenne pepper.

It is heavy, constipating.

Buttermilk is less mucus forming, with salt is prefered.

xi) Dairy products + whole grains + wheat, brown rice + Nourishing fruits - Banana, Pappaya + Complex Carbohydrates Potatoes.

xii) Sugar

Needed for body growth.

Jaggery - best form of sugar

Mapple syrup

Molases

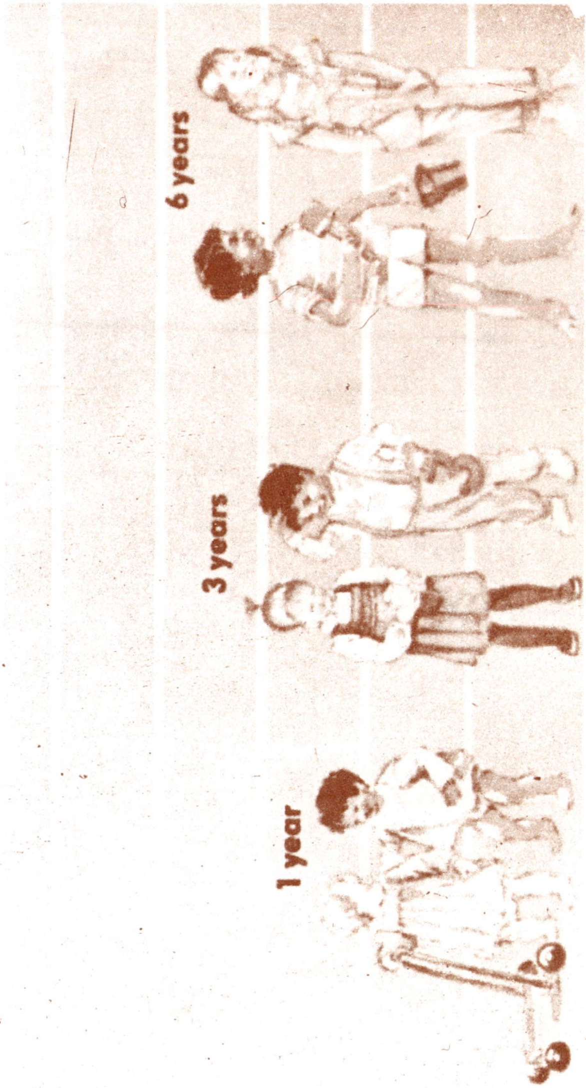
1 year
3 years
6 years

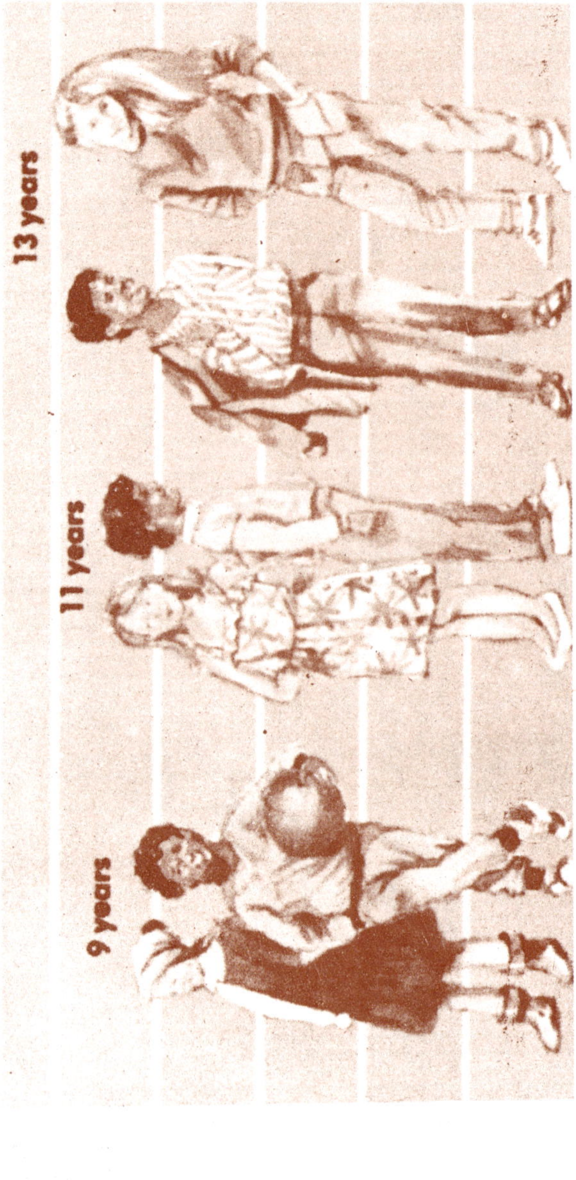
9 years
11 years
13 years

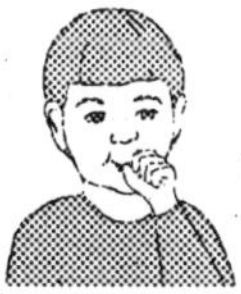

Rice/Barly malt

Unrefined sugar

xiii) Honey is concentrated sugar. Use in small amounts - as sweetener or medicine.

Good with herbs - Tonics, expectorants.

Flavouring agent. Enhances the effect.

Harder to digest as compared to sugar can even stimulate the paureace sugar cannot combine will with most of foods and causes gases/fermentation.

xiv) Raw sugar + Wholegrain or milk for children.

xv) Herbal confections - contain honey, ghee, nuts and tonic herbs.

3) Oils - Certain amount of oil is necessary in diet.

More in children for growth.

Oily food causes mucus and aggavates many childhood diseases.

Ghee, Sesame oil is best.

Ghee is easier for digest than oil.

Oil is useful for massage.

Warm oil massage calms nervous system, helps promote sleep, nourishes skin.

Increases child's feeling of being nurtured and cared for.

4) Spices

i) It regulate metabolism.

ii) Warm mildly sweet spices eg. Ginger, Cinamon, Cardmom, Coriander, Fennel are preferable.

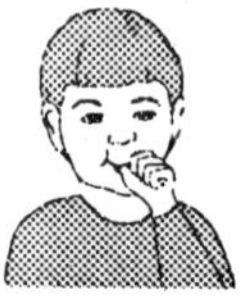

iii) Mild spices but not warm such as Turmuric, Cumin, Basil.

iv) Hot spices - Use carefully

Cayenne, Hot chillies, black pepper.

5) Herbs

Ashwagandha (Withania somnifera)
Shatavari (Asparagus racemosus)
Amalaki (Emblica officinalis)
Bala (Cida cordifolia)
} Energy tonics

Vacha (Calamus) - Increases intelligence

Brahmi (Gotukola) - Improves mind, cleanses blood, calms emotions.

Medicated ghee

Chavanprash - Growth food.

Brahmi Rasayan

6) Yoga

Meditation - Stories of Hanuman

Imaginative power be attuned to the symbols of cosmic mind.

6

Kalpani
(Paediatric preparations)

Liquids	No. of Ingredients	Action/use
1) Aravindasava (Lotuses, Draksha)	24	refreegerent
2) Balkadu (Balharitaki, Pippali, Shunthi)	09	Appetiser
3) Kumari Kalpa (Alovera, Dashamool)	28	Liver, cough
4) Medhamrita (Prasham) (Calamus, Bramhi, Jamatansi)	08	Memory & Tranquility
5) Abhayarishta (Haritaki, Shunthi, Draksha Corianders)	12	Constipation Hyperacidity
6) Kutajarishta (Kutaj, (Kumbhi bark)	04	Diarrhoea Dysentery Colitis
7) Vidangarishta (Embelia fruit, Trikatu, Indrayava)	13	Worms Digestive
8) Paripathadikwath (Paripatha, Guduchi, Bhunimb)(Phylanthus Nimb)	07	Fevers (Measals, chicken pox)
9) Chavanprash (Amalaki, Triphala, Dashmoola, Ashwagandha)	40	Debility, promotes defence system of body.

Liquids	No. of Ingredients	Action/use
10) Gulkand (Rose petals)	03	Burning sensation, after fever
11) Adulsa compound or Vasosin	06	Cough, Br. Asthama Laryngitis
12) Baljeevan (Shatavari, Rosebuds, Ashwagandha, pippali)	07	Tonic, prevent diseases
13) Dadimavleha (Pomgranate extract)	01	Diarrhoea, Dysentery, Cough
14) Krumihar (Wormol) (Drumstick plant Embelia fruits, worm seed Kirmani Ajwayan)	05	Worm infestation
15) Ajasthi Bhasma	01	Rickets weakness
16) Ativishadi churna (Atis long pepper, karkatshringi (Chinese gulls)	03	Vomiting, Fever cough
17) Krimi Kuthar (Trikatu, Indrayam, Palmirbeej)	22	Worms, fever, Vomitting
18) Krumimudgarasa (Vidang, Palashbeej, Karaskar)	06	Worms
19) Sanjeevani Guti (Vidanga, Shunthi, Bhallataka)	10	Teething trouble worms Diarrhea
20) Sookshma Triphala	04	Blood purifer

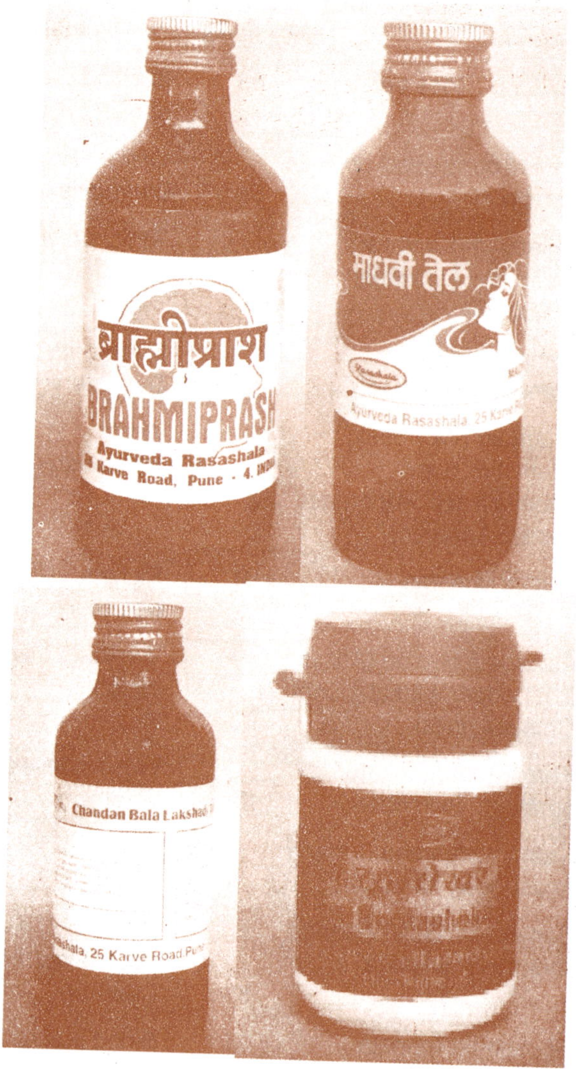
ब्राह्मीप्राश
BRAHMIPRASH
Ayurveda Rasashala
Karve Road, Pune - 4.
माधवी तेल
Ayurveda Rasashala
Chandan Bala
25 Karve Road

7

Scope of Kaumarbhritya (Paediatrics in Ayurveda)

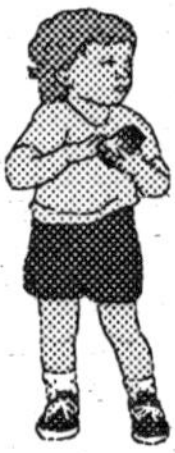

1) No branch of medicine is concerned so much with the growth and development of an individual as is 'Kaumarbhritya'. The nomenclature itself is self explanatory. Kumara : Bala

Growth pertains to physical or structural increase in size. Development pertains to functional or physiological increase in capacity.

In this branch i. e. the branch concerned with development of children. The other matters included are :

1) Ksheeradoshasanshodhan - Study of breast milk - its composition, qualities, impurities, remedies to purify it.

2) Dushtastanyasamutthanam Vyadhinam Upashamanartham - Treatment of disease caused by substandard or contaminated milk and major source of nutrition.

The main diet of the infant is milk and growth and development depends on it.

3) It also includes study of diseases caused by environmental factors especially the factors which behave as ghosts or demons (we may understand them now as bacteria & viruses). The children are vulnerable or special risk group and are very prone to attacks of diseases caused by these factors and hence a special mention of these diseases.

"Dushtagraha Samutthanam Vyadhinam Upashamanartham"

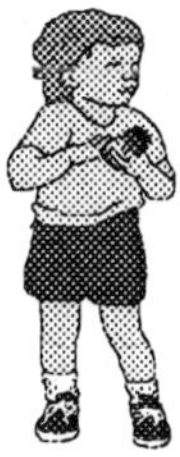

2) Ankur - Sapling

Though all the organs and tissues of the human body are destined to develop, the major portion of development occurs in first 5 years of life. Hence growth and development and for that matter, nutrition and protection are extremely important in a child.

In ancient texts, the child is compared to a Sapling just as (i) season (ii) soil (iii) water and (iv) seed are the four factors essential for germination of the seed into a sapling, so is the case in a human foetus and infant.

(i) Rutu i. e. season = Rutukala i. e. ovulation period.

(ii) Kshetra i. e. soil = Garbhashaya i. e. uterus.

Foetus -

(iii) Ambu i. e. water = Rasadhatu i. e. maternal blood.

(iv) Beeja i. e. Seed = Artava - Shukra

(i) Rutu - seasonal changes e. g. heat-cold.

(ii) Kshetra - Air and environment in which the child dwells.

Infant -

(iii) Ambu - Nutrition - milk and food

(iv) Beeja - Body.

Nutrition and protection are vital for survival, growth and development of a child. In case of diseases of children i. e. Bal Rogas, please see that nutrition is maintained all

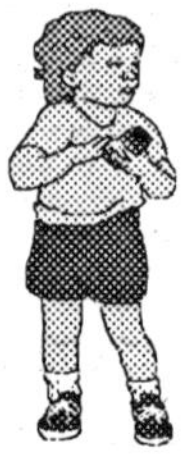

the time and that the child does not fall a pray or become a victim of the Grahas and Rakshas as lurking in the environment in the form of bacteria and viruses.

Thus Nutrition and Protection are the two main pillars which are essential for normal growth and development of a child.

Special Care :

The tissues and organs i. e. Dhatus and Avayavas are new and food and activities are so limited that Doshajanya Vikara i. e. metabolic diseases are not so common in children.

On the other hand because of delicate tissues (Soukumarya) less surface area (Alpakayatva) and because of not being accustomed or familiar to the new environment, Agantu diseases i. e. diseases caused by infection, trauma are more common in children.

Hold the child in such a way that it feels comfortable Gatrasukham Gruheeyata - Do not frighten Na Tarjayeta - Do not wake suddenly from sleep Sahasa Na Pratibodhayeta - Do not change the position suddenly; Do not make it sit unless it sits by itself and certainly not before 6 months.

Protect it from getting entangled in the clothes - Vastrapatat, from the contact of stranger - Parasparshat and from starvation - Langhanat.

Do not expose it to strong sunlight, heavy wind, too much dark or forests. Keep away from dirty places, unsupported

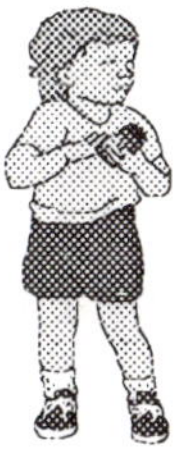

places, uneven places, dust, rain and smoke. Be pleasant and tender so that it becomes alert, healthy and happy.

Kumaragar (Child Room)

To ensure all this, Kumaragar, i. e. separate nursery or dwelling for children especially the new born and the infant is advocated.

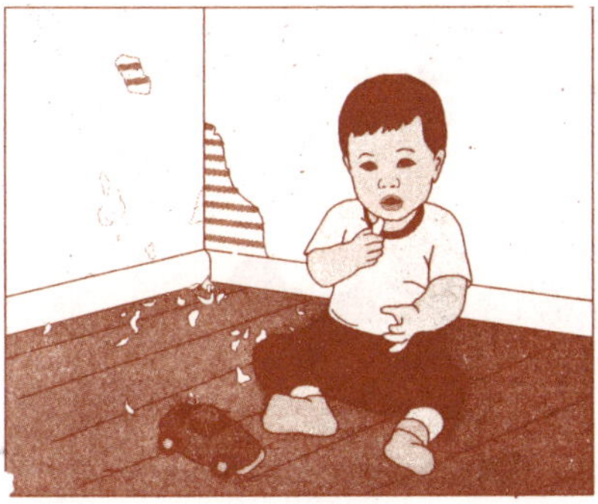

Specific guidlines are prescribed for the site, the building, direction, architecture, inner plan, water supply toilet, equipment, linen clothes and even the toys and the playground.

Rakshoghnavidhi for disinfection of air and clothes is advocated. Warnings are given to protect the child like a wounded man from flies, Krumi etc. Vranitopasneeya Upacharet.

a) Bhoomi i. e. ground should be Dhrudha i. e. firm and devoid of insects.

b) Vastu i. e. building should be Prashasta i. e. spacious. Architecture should be Ramya i. e. attractive, Not dark - Airy but no windy - well planned with separate Kitchen, water supply bathroom, toilet.

c) Rutusukham - equipped according to season.

d) Pravaran i. e. clothes

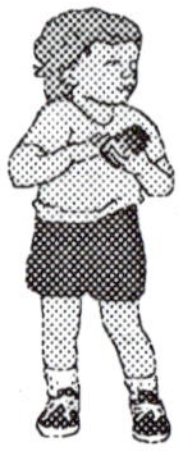

e) Mrudu - soft, Laghu - light, Shuchi - Clean, Sugandhi - Scented.

f) Shayana Astaran i. e. bed sheet linens

g) Suprakshalit - well washed, Shuddha - disinfected, Shushka - dried.

Disinfecting agents for funigation - Dhoopan are Brahmi, Jatamansi, Shwetadurva, Guggul, Vacha, Atasi, Hingu, Uda, Ajmoda.

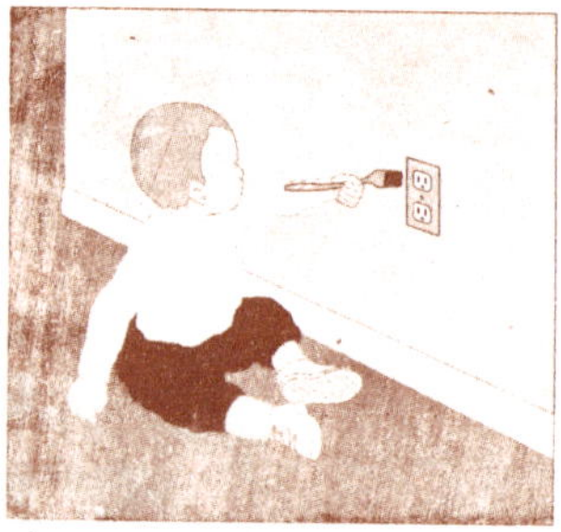

The toys should be

i) Vichitra - attractive

ii) Ghoshvali - Making sounds

iii) Abhiramani - pleasant

iv) Aguruni - light

v) Ateekshnagrani - without pointed or sharp ends

vi) Anasyapraveshani - cannot enter the mouth

vii) Avitrasanani - safe

viii) Play ground should be even, smooth, not studded with rough things like sand and stones. The ground should be clean and sprinkled with decoctions of Vacha, Pippali, Nimba etc.

ix) The home should be manned by caring people and attended by an experienced physician.

Nutrition

Thus it is evident that unimpaired nutrition and protection are very important factors for the growth and development

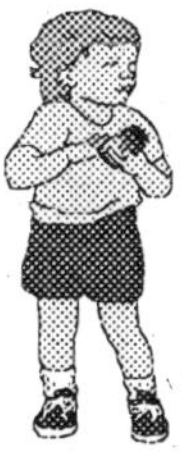

of a child. Nutrition in general and how to safeguard it while treating a disease in particular is very important. Malnutrition is one of the main causes of mortality and morbidity in children.

Praninam Punarmoolam Aharo - Food is the basis of a being, is very true of a child.

All the organs and the tissues especially the brain are developed in first 5 years.

Preenan : i. e. nourishment of these by the Ahar rasa i. e. digested and product of the food is very important. Milk and food provide these essential factors for the growth.

In case of an adult the tissues and organs are maintained (Dharayati) by Ahar rasa. But in case of a child they are both developed (Tarpayati Vardhayati) and maintained (Bharayati) by Ahar rasa.

On the basis of Ahar i. e. food intake, childhood has been divided into 3 stages.

1) Ksheerap - First year of life where milk is the main food.

2) Ksheerannad - Next two years Dwisanvatsarparaha where milk and food from main ingredients of diet.

3) Annad - After 3 years; where main ingredient is food.

Ksheer & Ksheerap Avastha

There is no substitue for mother's milk in the first six months. It appears that nature meant the human young ones to thrive on their mother's milk - Matureva.

This shows the importance of breast milk in the growth

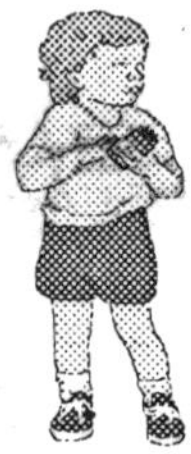

and development. It forms the main basis. That is why so much importance is given to study of milk and breast milk is highly advocated. A special Adhyay is allocated to study of milk, its quality, nutrient value, purity and so on.

The child is completely dependant upon the mother for feeding. The mental and social development of the child are also depedant upon the mother therefore Maternal health and care are also included in Kaumarbhritya Tantra.

Just as in the churning of oceans Gods got Nector, so in the body of the mother milk is produced which is like a nector to the infant.

It is the best restorative foremost in - Jeevaniya, Ksheero hi Sadyobalamadadati - quick restorative, Drudhikarotyashu Tathendriyani - reinforces the organs, Ojaso Varudhanam - increases vigour and resistance.

Stanya Sampat (Good breast milk)

The bresat milk is clean, sterile. It fully meets the requiremtns. It is available at the correct temperature. It does not require preparation or money. Suckling is good for the baby to develop jaws. It has bacteriostatic effect therefore it stays for a longer time.

Stanyasampat - Some physical properties of good pure milk are discribed :

i) Sheetal - having a particular temperature

ii) Amalam - clear, Tanu - Thin, Shankhabhasma - white as a shankha, Aphenilam - without froth, Atantumat - not

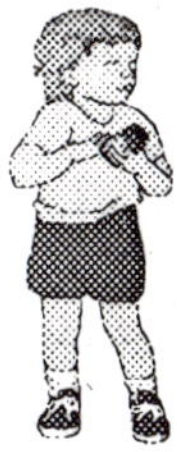

sticky, when instilled in water Apsunyastam. It should neither float nor sink.

iii) Na Upaplavate fNa Avaseedati - But should completely mix and become one with water - Ekeebhavam Gachhati.

iv) Thus in Ksheerap stage in first six months milk is the only diet.

v.) Oja, Teja - Vigour, resistance, immunity all are provided by breast milk.

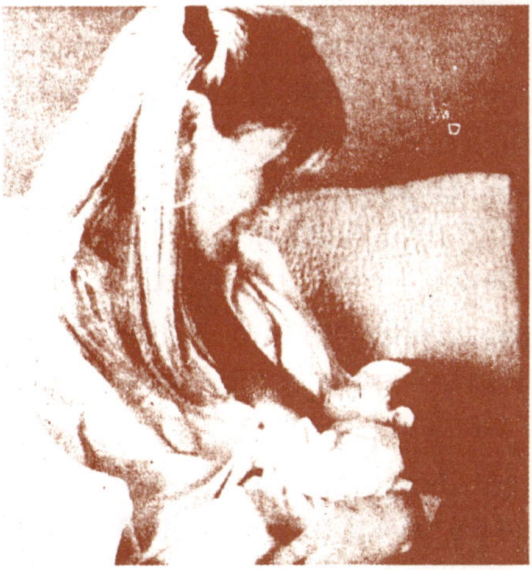

If the mother's milk is not available for some reason a Dhatri - should be employed or the milk of cow and goat somewhat resemble mother's milk.

Stanyabhave Payachhagam Gavyam wa Tadguṅam Pibet.

Annaprashan (Weaning)

In Ksheerap stage supplement by food has to be instituted from 6 months onwards. This is called 'weaning' or Annaprashan.

Shashthennaprashanam masi kramat taccha prayojate - It is a gradual process supplementing suitable solid food.

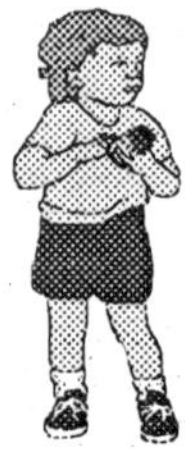

Bhajedyatha yatha chalam stanyam lyayam tatha taya.

As it starts taking solid food gradually the quantity of milk is reduced in that ration so that by the end of one year i. e. Ksheerap avastha. The child starts taking good amount of solid food, fruit juices Yoosha i. e. soups etc.

Thus it reaches the stage of Ksheerannad i. e. taking both milk and food.

When mother is not well breast milk may not be sufficient. It goes on crying even after feeding, does not sleep soundly - does not get good motion or profuse urine.

In such cases supplementary cow milk or goat milk should be given. It is treated by Brunhana drugs like Brahmi, Bala and sugar is added.

Usually vehicle for any medication in a child is Madhu (honey) and Ghruta (Ghee), in the form of Leha - paste. It may be nutrition or medication.

Food given to children should be Laghu i. e. easy for digestion and Brunhan i. e. giving energy (protein energy) and Ojovardhak i. e. increases immunity.

Fruit juices - Shalishashtika, Rice - Mudagayush, To promote Teja & Oja i. e. energy and resistance, Different Leha - pastes are advocated e. g. Suwarnaprasha - on a clean and washed stone little water is sprinkled. Gold shold be rubbed on it and a paste prepared by mixing honey and ghee.

It gives bala i. e. strength. It is beneficial, improves

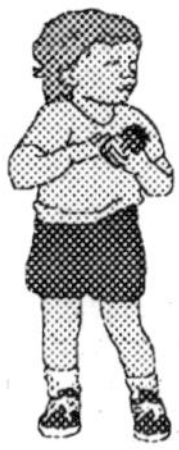

complexion and keeps away Grahas (by increasing resistance or immunity).

Brahmi Ghruta, Kalyanak Ghruta - Medhakar - (increases I. Q.), Abhaya ghruta - Rakshoghna - antiinfective, Sanvardhan Ghruta - for better development - in underweight children and in delayed mild stones.

Ksheerannad - (Milk and Food)

By the time the child enters this stage it has started taking solid food in good amount.

The food should be Laghu - light, easy for digestion by the tender alimentary canal. Brunhan i. e. giving energy - rich in protein, Madhur - sweet, Snigdha - soft, Sheeta - not hot, Hita - compatible.

The engery requirement of an year-old child is half the requiremtn of a young woman. This shows how essential it is to provide Brunhan and Ojovardhak food.

Dantodbhav (Teething)

By this time dentination also has started. There is irritation of the gums (Dantotsdha) - Kandu (itching). The child feels like biting - Yad Yad Alabhate - whatever it gets, Tad Tad Asyam Nayati. It tries to put in the mouth and bite. Special modak is crunchy balls are advocated for this. They are cruncy sweet. They satisfy the urge to bite and at the same time provide Laghu Brunhan ingradients rich in protein energy.

Main ingredients are Laja - pop corn - Guda - Sata - sugar, Satu - soya. They are meant for a child who is

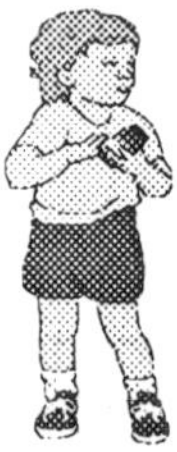

Apastanya who is being 'weaned' - taken away from breast feeding.

The other ingradients of these Modak are -

1) Preenan Modak - Nourishing, Priyalmajja madhuk madhu laja sitopalaiha

2) Deepan modak - Balabilwa ela sharkara laj saktu

3) Sangrahi modak - Dhatakipushpa sharkara laja tarpanaha.

The main ingredients are pop corn, Guda or sugar and soya and it is made crunchy. Other ingradients are added as per the need. If you want them to be more nourishing add nuts honey glycerizza. If you want them to be Deepan add cardamom, tender Bilwa, If you want them to be binding add Dhataki flowers.

Thus for the first three years one has to be very particular about even minor things. Nutrition and protection should be the guiding signals. Then the child grows to be Satwasampanna - intelligent, Prasannamana : happy and Niroga : i. e. healthy when it enters the annad stage.

Annad (Solid food)

When these things are observed the Annad stage passes on very smoothly giving scope for development of various faculties in the child.

8

Food as Medicine

1. CONSTIPATION (MALAVRODHA)

Constipation means no proper/ clear bowel action regularly. Difficulty in evacuation. Large intestine becomes sluggish. Irregular bowel habits. Irregular meals, to eat hurridly, faulty food habits are the causes of constipation. Worries, mental strain, fear, sedentary life are the causes of this disease. Purgatives and laxatives are harmful to the intestine.

1) HONEY is mild laxative. Without any trouble it clears the bowels. Due to its sweet taste children can eat very easily. It is useful for patients of any age and sex. 1-2 tea spoons 2-4 times/day.

2) MILK is best remedy for useful in constipation. Due to regular habit of milk drinking there will not be constipation at all.

3) SESAME SEEDS are useful in constipation. It may be used in food. (2-3 times per day).

4) APPLE is good known laxative. It is more useful when taken on empty stomach. (1/2-1 apple a day).

5) Well riped BANANA is mild laxative and it is useful (1-2 per day).

6) Eat one CUCUMBER for clean bowel action every day.

7) DATES are useful in constipation. Eat 2-5 dates a day.

8) FIG eating is good. Without straining, bowels are cleared. Fig syrup is also used. Eat 2-4 figs a day.

9) GRAPES are good for combating the constipation. It contains acidic substance, which produces more peristaltic movements of the intestine.

10) Fresh GUAVA to be eaten 1/2-1 a day which are useful.

11) LEMON JUICE 1-2 tea spoons with a cup of warm/ plain water in the morning is remedy for constipation.

12) Include MANGO in diet whenever possible. It reduces constipation

13) MUSKMELON is useful in constipation. Eat it.

14) Eat 1 MANDRIN in the morning and at night. Constipation will be cured.

15) RASINS/SULTANAS are known as laxatives. It contains cellulose, which promotes good peristalsis of the intestine.

16) TOMATOS are mild laxatives. Eat riped tomatos. Useful in constipation.

17) COCONUT MILK/WATER is very mild laxative, can be used in constipation.

18) Use in your diet WHEAT with HUSK, BROWN RICE, PULSES, PEANUTS, LIVER, MUTTON it is remedy for constipation.

19) Fruits with skin, steamed vegetables, bread of grains, contains vit. B-1 and hence are useful in constipation.

20) 1/2 cup ofYOGHURT/CURD add 1 tea spoon of sugar, drink it two times a day. It is useful in constipation.

21) 1/2 glass of BUTTER MILK add 1 tea spoon of sugar

and drink it 2 times a day for curing constipation.

22) Eat BEAT every day. There will be no constipation.

23) Eat roasted POTATO every day it cures constipation.

24) Eat RADISH which is useful in constipation.

25) Use BARLEY in diet it is useful in constipation.

26) 1 Tea spoon of GHEE and cup of WARM MILK at bed time relieves constipation.

27) Masha (Kidney bean) is good remedy.

2) DIARRHOEA (ATISAAR)

Loosenes of the bowels. Sometimes peristalsis of the intestine are increased hence one may get loose motions several times a day. Bacteria, viruses etc. enter our body through food, water etc. If there is inflamation of the inner coating of intestine, due to intestinal worms, some drugs, psychological disturbance are the causes of diarrhoea.

1) APPLE contains pectin. It is useful in controlling the loose motions. Children are more benefitted. Give them 1 to 4 teaspoons of pulp of sweet and riped apple. It controls diarrhoea within 2 days. It is also helpful in habit of loose motions. It is controlled. Apple juice is disinfectant for stomach and intestine. It prevents bacterias etc.

2) Raw BANANA is astringent. Mucus membrane of intestine is contracted by intake of this type of banana.

3) GRAPES are also useful.

4) Raw PINEAPPLE is also useful.

5) COCONUT milk/water is also useful in loose motions, Cholera and similar conditions.

6) CARROT is dis-infectant hence useful in controlling the diarrhoea.

7) GARLIC has the same utility.

8) Plenty of WATER is to be drunk for any type of diarrhoea, it replaces the loss of body fluid.

9) If diarrhoea is due to be deficiency of niacin then one can include peanuts, PULSES, unpolished or brown RICE and WHEAT in his/her diet.

10) Drink BUTTER MILK, TEA and COFFEE.

11) Boiled MILK is useful but raw milk may cause loose motions.

12) BARLEY water, WHEAT, water of white of egg, corn flower, Araroot, Ricewater, Brandy, Sherry are useful in acute diarrhoea.

13) Use BUTTER MILK, Tea, Coffee, Red wine, Wharterbery wine in chronic diarrhoea.

14) Soup of PULSES is useful in any type.

15) POPCORN water and ghee are useful in any type.

16) Eat YOGHURT or curds if diarrhoea is often.

17) Drink MOLASSES and eat sprouted WHEAT.

3. GROWTH : BODY AND HEIGHT

Growth in size and length of a living being means body growth.

Height and weight is especially more at the time of puberty means for Age 14 to 18 years.

1) Include BUTTER in the every day diet. Height will be more. It contains 80% fat and vit. A & D.

2) BANANA with brown spots on the skin is riped one and best. Give it to children. It is easy for digestion and good for body growth.

3) MANDRINE to be eaten. It is useful in height increasing. 4 tea spoons to 1 cup of orange juice according to age may be given.

4) PEAS are best for growth. It contains superior quality proteins.

5) SOYABEAN or its milk is very useful for body growth.

6) Slow growth of body or less height, it may be due to deficiency of proteins. PULSES, PEANUTS, EGGS, MILK and fish are to be included in diet, for rich supply of proteins.

7) Calcium is necessary for body health and growth. Hence drink milk, pulses, sesame seeds, corriander seeds, fish etc.

8) Drink more WATER. It is useful.

9) RAGI grains (Elucine Coracana) to be given to children for proper and good growth.

4) INDIGESTION

Also known as Dyspepsia. No proper digestion of food then it is known as indigestion. This is not a disease. It is a symptom one can see in many diseases. Errors and irregularities in eating and drinking causes Dyspepsia e.g. to eat on and off, to eat more than required due to habit, to eat hurriedly etc..

Feeling heaviness in abdomen, pain in abdomen, nausea, vomiting, headache are symptoms in Dyspepsia.

1) Take 2 teaspoons of HONEY 3-4 times a day, as honey does not ferment. It is very useful in indigestion.

2) BANANA is best food. If indigestion is due to carbohydrets eat banana 1-3 times a day, as per your taste. It will be useful for you.

3) GRAPES are light for digestion. Hence can be used liberally. Those having delicate digestion – est 2-4 times a day.

4) Use LEMON juice 2-4 times a day before or after food. It produces more saliva in mouth and stomach (i.e. gastric juice). Hence good for digestion.

5) Take ORANGE juice for curing indigestion. It produces more digestive juices.

6) PINAPPLE is good for digestion. Eat after food. It get rid complaints of digestion.

7) When nothing is digested then take POMGRANATE. It is easy for digestion.

8) Drink COCONUT WATER (milk) for gases in stomach. Take a glass of it three hours after taking food.

9) GARLIC is useful in gases in stomach, discomfort in abdomen.

5) PYREXIA (FEVER) (JWARA)

Fever or pyrexia means rise in body temperature. When there is increase in body temperature metabolic action is also increases. (Anabolic and katabolic action). Due to this increased metabolic action more carbohydrates, proteins and fluid is expelled out of body. Sodium chloride is also destroyed.

Due to increase in heat in our surroundings. Entry of bacteria in our body, more loss of fluid from our body, inflammation, infection or trauma to brain are various reasons of fever.

1) There is no proper digestion in any fever. In such condition it is necessary without taxing digestive system energy of the body is to be maintained, and in such condition HONEY is very useful. Take honey 3-4 times a day 2-4 spoons at a time. It is more useful in pneumonia and typhoid.

2) There is destruction of proteins in the fever. Hence it is necessary to compensate the loss of proteins and supply all constituents to the body. CANE SUGAR juice is the best.

3) GRAPE SUGAR is very easily assimilable in the blood hence as a food in fever grapes be utilized.

4) ORANGES are good in any fever. Its juice is useful for body nutrition. It is also very easy for digestion and there is no normal digestion in fevers, hence use in fevers.

5) Soak SULTANA (RAISIN) in warm/cold water for twelve hours. Then this water be utilized for drinking in fever

cases. It is very useful.

6) Boil the water, then cool it and use for drinking in patients suffering from fever.

7) BUTTER MILK, COCONUT MILK/water and LEMON are useful in fever.

Soup of pulses may be given.

6. SKIN DISEASES (TWAKVIKARA)

Whole body is covered by the skin. Extensive area is exposed to the surroundings. Skin diseases are difficult to cure and treat. Sometimes there are chronic diseases. These diseases become obstacles to health and also interferes with the body beauty. Hence person concerned worries, and due to worry/tension skin diseases are aggravated.

1) HONEY is very useful in many skin diseases.

2) FIG is useful. Use plenty for eating.

3) GRAPES are very useful in many diseased conditions of the skin.

4) MANGO is useful for giving good luster of skin or blossoming the skin.

5) MUSK MELON is best in cases of eczema. If one lives on musk melon for 40 days continuously then this disease gets cured. There are many such examples. Hence eat musk melon.

6) SOYABIN is useful in curing fissures on the skin e.g. fissured eczema. Soyabin is good for maintaining the skin

health.

7) If skin is of dry type then use OILS, GHEE, PEANUTS in the diet. It relieves such complaints.

8) In this condition eat green VEGETABLES, MANGO, CARROT, LIVER etc. there will be good result.

9) In deficiency of riboflavin skin becomes dry. Use LIVER, MILK, PULSES, GREEN VEGETABLES, in your diet. One gets relief.

10) In deficiency of niacin there is itching of the skin, and it turns red. For such condition eat PULSES, PEANUTS, BROWN RICE, WHEAT etc.

11) For proper maintenance of skin, GRAINS, PULSES, LIVER and egg to be consumed daily.

There are wrinkles on the skin sometimes. It is due to loss of fluid and salt from the body, excessive sweating, diarrhoea, vomitting are other causes. For relieving such condition drink common salt mixed water sip by sip many times a day.

If eczema or wounds on skin are weeping or with more secretions then do not consume salt.

If skin is dry, rough and with pruritus then to get rid of this condition eat CABBAGE or Drink 50-175 ml. of juice of Cabbage.

7) VOMITING (CHHARDI)

A substance from the stomach if expelled out through mouth is known as vomiting. Entry of poisonous substances into the stomach, some drugs, in some

Fevers, Intestinal worms are the causes of vomiting.

1) In case of persistant vomiting and nothing is retained in the stomach, in such case patient is exhausted, becomes debilitated, then give HONEY 2 spoons 4-8 times a day as it is or with water. Energy / strength of body is retained and increases slowly.

2) Use LEMON. Gastritis will be reduced. Peristalsis of stomach becomes less and by that frequency of vomiting is reduced. Though lemon is acidic in nature it transforms into alkaline substance.

3) MANGO is good remedy for vomiting.

4) Drink COCONUT MILK / WATER for stopping the vomiting. It is better when other attempts have been failed.

5) Eat Ice for controlling the vomiting.

6) Preparing a mixture of LEMON, water and white of egg. Drink it. Good for relief in vomiting.

7) Mix one spoon of Brandy, Schampane and sparkling soda and drink it. It stops vomiting.

8) Aerated waters are useful.

9) Drink plenty of water sip by sip. It is useful.

10) Put some common salt on the tongue. It helps to stop the vomiting.

11) Grapes are useful in case of vomiting.

12) Lemon juice 2 spoons and a glass of water this mixture is to be taken for relief in case of vomiting.

13) A cup of milk and ½ spoon of soda-bi-carb powder.

8) WEIGHT GAIN (BRUMHANA)

Our body weight should be according to / related to the height of the body. If there is loss of weight, there might be some ailment in the body. People are taking many tonic preparations for gaining the weight. There should be proper nutrition of muscle tissues, smooth working of all organs of the body is essential. To have proper or suitable weight is essential for health and for good appearance also.

1) SUGAR CANE juice contains essential nutrient constituents, hence its use in weight gaining is useful.

2) MILK CREAM contains plenty of fatty substances. It also contains other useful constituents for body growth. Hence it is useful in gaining body weight.

3) MILK is useful for increasing body weight. Take 200 ml. milk every half an hour, do not eat anything. Take complete rest. One can gain half kg. Weight every day by this procedure.

4) EGGS are best for weight gain. Proteins and fats in it are useful for nutrition and growth for different body cells. Hence growth of total body and rise in body weight.

5) FISH is good for nutrition, growth and weight gain of body. Aminoacids contained in it are more useful. Fish is easy for digestion. Fish liver oir contains vit. A & D which is useful.

6) BUTTER is light for digestion and useful in this condition.

Take BANANAS and milk daily. It is a complete food.

9

Treatment of Diseases

(Dose mentioned is for adult. Give 1/3rd dose for Children)

1. Abdominal Colic / Pain in abdomen (Udarshool)

Introduction : Causes -

Indigestion, Acidity problems, Liver disorders, intestinal parasites, kidney disorders, inflammation, diseases of uterus and ovaries in females.

1) Choorna (Powder) :
   - **Eladi choorna** 1-3 gms with honey 3-4 times a day.

2) Gutivati (Tablets) :
   - **Lashunadivati** 250 mgms 3-4 times a day with warm water.
   - **Vatagajankusha** 125 mgms -250 mgms with warm water 3 times a day.

3) Asava (medicated wine) :
   - **Kanakasava** 10-20 ml with water after food.

4) Paka (syrup - Avaleha) :
   - **Lashunpak** 5-10 ml with warm water 3 times a day.

5) Ghruta (ghee) :
   - **Shatavarighruta** 10-20 mgms with milk 3 times a day.
   - **Tiktaka ghruta** 10-20 ml with milk 3 times a day.

6) Tail (oil) -
   - **Lakshaditail :** For external application to abdomen.

7) Lepa (paste) :

- **Darushataklep** application on abdomen.

8) Bhasma (Calx) :

- **Kapardik bhasma** 250-500 mgms 3 times a day with lemon juice or warm water.
- **Shankhbhasma** 500 mgms to 1 gm with warm water or lemon juice 3 times a day.

2. Allergy (Sheetapitta)

Introduction :

Intollerance to food, smell, environment, dust are described as allergy. Urticaria, redwheels appear on the skin.

1) Choorna (Powders) :

- **Avipattikarchoorna** 2-3 gms. with warm water.
- **Haridrakhandchoorna** 3-6 gms. with water after food.
- **Panchnimbachoorna** 250 - 500 mgms. with honey 3 times a day.
- **Triphala choorna** 1-2 gms 2 times with warm water

2) Guti/Vati (Tablets) :

- **Suvarnasootashekhar** 1 tablet 3 times a day.
- **Anticol (Pittashamak)** 2 tablets 3 times a day.
- **ACP Tabs** 2 tablet 3 times a day.
- **SSS 3 x - 1** tablet 3 times a day.

3) Asava (Medicated wines) :

Bhallatakasava 10-20 ml. with water 2 times after food.

4) Kwatha (decoction) :

- **Bhunimbadi Kwath** 10-20 ml. with water 2 times a day.
- **Paripathadikwath** 10-20 ml with water 2 times a day.

5) Phant (Tea)

- **BNK :** 2-3 times a day

3. Anaemia (Panduroga)

Introduction :

Quantity or quality of blood is reduced is known as Anaemia (Pandurog). Pallor is main symptom. Debility, irritability are other symptoms.

1) Choorna (Powders) :

- **Navayasa choorna** 1gm-2gms 3 times a day with ghee & sugar.

2) Guti/Vati (Tablets) :

Arogyavardhini - 2 tablets (each 125 mgm) 3 times a day with water.

3) Asava (Medicated wines) :

- **Punarnavasava** 10-20 ml 2 times after food with equal amount of water.
- **Lohasva** 10-20 ml 2 times after food with water.

4) Arishta : (Medicated wines) :

- **Punarnavadyarishta** 10-20 ml with water after food.
- **Rohitakarishta** 10-20 ml with water after food.

5) Kwatha (decoction) :

Punarvadikwath 10-20 ml. after food 2 times a day with water.

6) Avaleha (Jam) :

Dadimavleha 10-20 ml 3 times a day.

7) Ghruta (Ghee) :

Tiktakaghruta 10-20 ml 3 times a day with milk.

Dadimadighruta 10-20 ml 3 times a day with milk.

8) Bhasma (Calx / Ash) :

- **Abhrakbhasma** 125 mgms - 250 mgms 3 times a day with honey.
- **Kasisbhasma** 125 mgms - 250 mgms 3 times a day with ghee or honey.
- **Kantaloha** 125 mgms - 250 mgms 3 times a day with honey or ghee.
- **Tamrabhasma** 50 mgms - 100 mgms 3 times a day with honey.
- **Mandurbhasma** 125 mgms - 250 mgms 3 times a day with honey or ghee.
- **Roupyabhasma** 125 mgms - 250 mgms 3 times a day with honey.
- **Lohabhasma** 125 mgms - 250 mgms 3 times per day with honey or ghee.

- **Suvarnamakshikbhasma** 250 mgms - 500 mgms 3 times per day with honey or ghee.

❑ **Other Products :**

- **Tapyadiloha** 250 mgms - 500 mgms 3 times a day with honey or ghee.
- **Navayasloha** 125 mgms - 250 mgms 3 times per day with honey or ghee.

9) Rasakalpa (with mercury) :

- **Panchamrutaparpati** 125 mgms - 250 mgms with ghee or sugar 3 times a day
- **Lohaparpati** 125 mgms - 250 mgms 3 times a day with ghee or sugar 3 times.
- **Panduroga tablets** 1 tablet 3 times a day with food.

10) Phant (Tea)

- **ASforte** 2 times a day.

4. Anorexia (Agnimandya)

Introduction :

Agni is responsible for conversion of food into suitable substance to nourish tissues of body. Mand Agni (low fire) is cause of all diseases. Anorexia (loss of appetite) is main sympton.

1) Choorna (Powders) :

- **Lavanabhaskar Choorna** - 1-3 gms with butter milk or warm water.
- **Ashtanglavana Churna** - 2-3 gms after food & water.

- **Chitrakadi Choorna** - 1-2 gms 3 times a day with water.

2) Guti/Vati (Tablets) :

- **AgnitundiRasa** 125 mgms Tablet 1-2, three times a day with warm water.
- **Lashunadivati** 250 mgms Tablet. One tablet 3-4 times a day.

3) Asava (Medicated wine) :

- **Panchakolasava** - 10-20 ml with equal amount of water two times a day after food.

4) Arishta (Medicated wine) :

- **Jeerakadyarishta** - 10-20 ml with equal amount of water after food two times a day.

5) Avaleha (Jam) :

- **Bharangiavaleha** - 10-20 ml. with luke warm water 3 times a day.

6) Ghruta (Ghee) :

- **Tikatakaghruta** 1-2 gms with warm milk 3 times a day.
- **Shatpalaghruta** 10-20 ml two times a day with warm water.

7) Paka (Candy) :

- **Lashunapaka** 1-2 gms 3 times a day with lukewarm water.

8) Bhasma (Calx / Ash) :

- **Kapardikbhasma** - 250 mgms to 500 mgms two times a day with lemon juice or buttermilk or lukewarm water.

9) Other :

- TKT Tablets 1-2 tablets 3 times before food.

10) Phant (Tea)

- **TKT** 2 times a day before meals.

5. Asthma (Bronchial) (Tamakshwasa)

Introduction :

Difficulty in breathing. Children & young people are more vulnerable. Males are more prone for Bronchial Asthma.

1) Choorna (Powders) :

- **Karpuradi choorna** : 2-3 gms. with honey or warm water 3 times a day.
- **Pipalyadi choorna** : 2-3 gms. with honey or warm water 3 times a day.
- **Yashtimadhu choorna** 2-3 gms. with honey 3-4 times a day.

2) Gutivati (Tablets)

- **Bruhatvata chintamani** 50 mgms with honey or ginger juice 3 times a day.
- **Hemagarbha tablet** - 1 tablet 3 times a day with warm water.
- **Hirakbhasma tablet** 1 tablet 3·times a day with warm water.
- **Suvarnamalini vasant** 125 mgms with sugar and butter.

3) Asava (Medicated wine) :

- **Kanakasava** : 5 ml. with warm water every half hour till attack subsides.

4) Arishta (medicated wine) :

- **Dashamularista** 10-20 ml. with water after meals 2 times a day.

5) Avaleha (jam) (syrup) :

- **Ardrakavleha** - 5-10 ml./gms. with water four times a day.
- **Chavanprashavleha** 1-2 teaspoonful 2 times a day.
- **Vasavleha** 1/2 teaspoonful 2 times a day.
- **Vasosin** 2 teaspoonfuls 3-4 times a day.

6) Tail (Oil) :

Narayan oil 5 ml. warm oraly to subside the attack of breathlessness.

7) Bhasma (Calx) :

- **Abhrak bhasma** 125-250 mgms with honey 3 times a day.
- **Manikyarasa** 50 to 100 mgms with honey 3 times a day.
- **Shrungbhasma** 250-500 mgms with honey 3 times a day.

8) Rasakalpa :

- **Makardhwaja** 25-50 mgms with honey 3 times a day.
- **Sameerpannag** 30-50 mgms with honey 3 times a day.
- **Suvarnarasasindoor** 25-50 mgms with honey 3 times a day.

9) Phant (Tea)

- **TKT** 2-4 times a day.

6. Common Cold (Nasopharyngitis) (Pratishyay)

Introduction :

Nasal secretions, running nose, sneezing, headache, mild fever are the symptoms of Nasopharyngitis. Accumulation of aam (half digested food material) or allergy to dust, viral infection are the common causes.

1) Gutivati (Tablets) :

- **Nagguti** 125 mgms 3 times with honey or warm water.
- **Sanjeevani guti** 250-500 mgms 2 times after food with water.
- **Tribhuvanakeerti** 250 mgms with honey 3 times a day.

2) Avaleha :

- **Ardrakavleha** 5-10 ml. with water 3-4 times a day.
- **Kantakaryavleha** 10-20 ml. with warm water 3 times a day.
- **Vasosin** 5-10 ml. 4 times a day.

3) Tail (Oil) : for Nasya (Nasal administration)

- **Anutail** 1-2 drops in nose 2-3 times / day.
- **Shadbindutail** 1-2 drops in nose 2-3 times/day.
- **Vachatail** 1-2 drops in nose 2-3 times / day.

4) Phant (Tea)

- **TKT** 2-3 times a day.

7. Constipation (Malavrodha)

Introduction :

No proper or regular bowel movements. Straining or hard scabela may be few of symptoms.

1) Choorna (Powders) :

- **Avipattikar choorna** 2-3 gms with warm water at bed time.
- **Gandharvaharitaki choorna** 2-3 gms with warm water at bed time.
- **Triphala choorna** 2-3 gms with warm water 3 times a day.
- **Sukhasarak choorna** 2-3 gms with warm water at bed time.

2) Gutivati (Tablets) :

- **Arogyavardhini** 500 mgm. with warm water 2 times a day.
- **Sukhasarakvati** 1 gm with warm water at bed time & in the morning.
- **Icchabhedi** 125 mg. of bed time with warm water.

3) Asava (Medicated wine) :

Drakshasava 20 ml. with water after food.

4) Arishta (Medicated wine) :

Abhayarishta 20 ml. with water 2 times a day.]

5) Phant (Tea)

- **HSG** 2 times a day.

8. Cough (Kasa)

Introduction :

It is a symptom in many diseases as well is a disease. Diseases of lungs, heart, throat problems & psychological disorders. Air inhaled with force & exhaled with force & noise known as cough.

1) Choorna (Powders) :

- **Dadimadi choorna** 2-4 gms with honey 3-4 times a day.
- **Karpuradi choorna** 2-3 gms with honey or water 3 times a day.
- **Sitopaladi choorna** 1-2 gms with milk or water 3 times a day.

2) Guti / Vati (Tablets)

- **Lavangadivati** 2 tablets 3-4 times a day for chewing (Tab. Cozenges).
- **Sookshma triphala** 1-2 tablets 3 times a day.
- **Tab** V 1-2 tablets 3 times a day.

3) Asava (Medicated wine) :

- **Drakshasava** 10-20 ml. with water after food. 2 times/ day.
- **Punarnavavasa** 10-20 ml. with water after food 2 times a day.

4) Avaleha (Jam) :

- **Ardrakavleha** 5-10 ml. 3-4 times a day.
- **Chavanprashavleha** 3-5 gms with milk 3 times a day.
- **Vasavleha** 5-10 gms 3 times a day.

- **Vasosin** 10 ml 3-4 times a day.

5) Ghruta (Ghee) :

   Vasaghruta 1 to 2 teaspoons with milk 3 times a day.

6) Bhasma (Calx / Ash) :

- **Kasis Bhasma** 125-250 mgms. with honey 3 times a day.
- **Shrungbhasma** 250-500 mgms. with honey 3 times a day.

7) Nasya (Nasal administration) :

   Anu Taila apply to nasal mucosa morning, evening with finger or cotton bud.

8) Ahar (Diet/Food) :

   Avoid cold, oily, more quantity of food.

9) Vihar (Movements) :

   Avoid exposure to cold.

10) Phant (Tea)

- **TKT** 2-3 times a day.

9. Debility / Weakness / Lassitude (Dourbalya)

Introduction :

Loss of body weight, Breathlessness, unable to carryout usual duties, low immunity.

1) Choorna (Powder) :

- **Ashwagandhadi choorna** 2-3 gms. with milk 3 times a day.

- **Shatavari kalpa** 1 teaspoon with milk 3 times a day.

2) Guti/Vati (Tablets) :

- **Tab ASplus** 1 tablet 2 times a day.

3) Asava (Medicated wine) :

- **Drakshasava** 10-20 ml. with water 2-3 times a day.

4) Arishta (Medicated wine) :

- **Ashwagandharishta** 10-20 ml. with water after meals.
- **Balarishta** 10-20 ml. with water after food 2 times a day.

5) Avaleha (Jam) :

Raktavardhak 1/2 teaspoonful 2 times with food.

6) Phant (Tea)

- **ASforte** 2 times a day.

7) **Tab Heerakbhasma** 1 tablets 2 times a day.

8) **Tab Hemagarbha** 1 tablet 2 times a day.

10. Diarrhoea (Loose Motions) (Atisaara).

Introduction :

Watery stools more times a day. Pain in abdomen, flatulence, indigestion are symptoms.

1) Choorna (Powders) :

- **Jatiphaladi choorna** 2-3 gms 3-4 times a day with buttermilk or water.
- **Dhanya panchak Choorna** 2-3 gms with honey after food.

- **Lavangadi choorna** 2-3 gms with honey or water 3 times a day.

2) Guti / Vati (Tablets) :

- **Sanjeevaniguti** 250 mgms 3-4 times a day with water.
- **Shankhodar** 125 mgms to 250 mgms 2-4 times a day with water or butter milk.

3) Asava (Medicated wines) :

- **Bhallatakasava** 10-20 ml. with water after food, two times a day.

4) Arishta (Medicated wines) :

- **Kutajarishta** 10-20 ml. with water 2 times/day after food.
- **Jeerakadyarishta** 10-20 ml. with water after food 2 times a day.
- **Babbulaydiarishta** 10-20 ml. with water after food.

5) Kwatha (decoction) :

- **Shatavaryadi kwath** 10-20 ml. with water 3 times a day.

6) Avaleha (Jam) :

- **Kutajavleha** 10-20 ml. 3-4 times a day with water.
- **Bilvavleha** 10-20 ml. 3 times a day with water.

7) Bhasma (Calx / Ash) :

- **Shankhbhasma** 500 mgms to 1 gm. 3 times a day.

8) Rasakalpa (with mercury) :

- **Rasaparpati** 125 mgms to 250 mgms 3 times a day with ghee & sugar.

- **Lokanathrasa** 250 mgms to 500 mgms 3 times a day with ghee & sugar.

9) Snehana (Oil) :

- **Chukrataila** 20-30 drops with warm water 3 times a day.

10) Phant (Tea)

- **JDA** 2-4 times a day.

11. Eczema

Introduction :

Swelling, inflamation of skin, (redness) pustules, Dry or Wet variety. Thickened skin. May be pruritus, burning sensation.

1) Choorna (Powders) :

- **Panchnimba choorna** 250-500 mgmsss with honey 3 times a day.

2) Guti / Vati (Tablets) :

- **Tab. D.C.** 1 tablet 3 times with water.
- **Gandhakrasayan** 500 mgm. to 1 gms. with water or honey 3 times a day.
- **Sookshma Triphala** 2 tablets 2-3 times a day.
- **Swayambhuva guggulu** 1 gm to 2 gms. with water 3 times a day.

3) Asava (Medicated wines) :

- **Sarivadyasava** 10-20 ml. with water 2 times a day.

4) Arishta (Medicated wines) :

- **Khadirarishta** 10-20 ml. with water 2 times a day.

5) Kwatha (decoction) :

- **Mahamanjishthadi Kwatha** - 10-20 ml. with water 2 times a day.

6) Bhasma (Calx / Ash) :

- **Vangbhasma** 250-500 mgms. with honey or milk 3 times a day.

7) Snehana (Oil) :

- **Vranashodhana Tail** - for external application.
- **Sahachar Tail** - for external application.

8) Phant (Tea)

- **DC** 2-3 times a day.

O

12. Epilepsy (Apasmar)

Introduction :

Epileptic fits occur. Broth to the mouth of a patiant. Heriditary problems. May be injury to Brain.

1) Guti/Vati (Tablets) :

- **Smrutisagar rasa** 125 mgm - 250 mgms 3 times a day with ghee.
- **Unmadgajakesari** 250 mgms to 500 mgms 3 times a day with ghee & sugar.
- **Bhutbhairav rasa** 250 mgms to 1 gm. 3 times a day with water.
- **Heerak Bhasmavati** (SP) vajra 1 tablet 3 times a day.

2) Arishta (Medicated wines) :

- **Saraswatarishta** 10-20 ml. with water 3 times a day.
- **Hemagarbha** tablet 1 tablet 3 times a day.

3) Avaleha (Jam) :

- **Abhayamalakiavaleha** 1 teaspoon with water 2 times a day.
- **Bramhiprash** 5-10 ml. with water 3 times a day.
- **Shankhapushpiavaleha** 10-20 ml. with water 3 times a day.

4) Ghruta (Ghee) :

- **Saraswatghruta** 10-20 gms with milk 3 times a day.
- **Kalyanak ghruta** 10-20 gms with milk 3 times a day.

5) Paka (Candu) :

- **Chopachini pak** 5-10 ml. with milk 3 times a day.

6) Snehana (Oil) :

- **Balatail** 5-10 ml. with milk 2 times a day.
- **Lakshadi Tail** massage to scalp 2 times a day.
- **Vacha Tail** for external application/Nasal administration.

7) Phant (Tea) :

- **AYT** Every 3 hours per day.

8) Nasya (Nasal administration) :

- **Panchgavyaghruta** 5-10 drops in nose.

9) Pishti :

- **Akik pishti** 125 mgms - 250 mgms with honey 3 times a day.

13. Fever (Jwar)

Introduction :

Body temperatures rises above normal is fever or pyrexia. Symptoms are as follows : (i) Face red & hot (ii) Dry Skin (iii) Loss of appetite (iv) Headache (v) Nausia or vommiting (vi) Constipation or loose motion (vii) Bodyache (viii) Yellow & less amount of urine (ix) Convulsions may appear in children.

1) Choorna (Powders) :

- **Mahasudarshan Choorna** 2 to 3 gms with honey 3 times a day.
- **Sitopaladi choorna** 1-2 gms with honey or water 3 times a day.

2) Guti/Vati (Tablets) :

- **MSK** Tablets 1-2 tablets 3 times a day with water.
- **Parijatak guti** 2 tablets 3 times a day with water.
- **Sanjeevaniguti** 2 tablets 3 times a day with water.
- **Suvarnasootashekharvati** 1 tablet 3 times a day with water.
- **Tribhuvana keerti** 1-2 tablets 3 times a day with water.

3) Arishta (medicated wine) :

- **Amrutarishta** 10-20 ml. with water after food 2 times a day.

4) Kwatha (decoction) :

- **Mahasudarshan Kwatha** 10-20 ml. with water 2 times a day.
- **Tiktapanchak kwatha** 10-20 ml. with water 3 times a day.

5) Ghruta (Ghee) :

- **Kalyanak ghruta** 1 to 2 tsp with milk 3 times a day.

6) Tail (Oil) :

- **Lakshadi tail** for external application to reduce the fever.

7) Bhasma :

- **Kamadudha** 250-500 mgm with honey 3 times a day.
- **Praval bhasma** 250-500 mgm with water 3 times a day.
- **Mouktika bhasma** 125-250 mgm with water 3 times a day.

8) Pishti :

- **Jaharmohara pishti** 250-500 mgm with honey 3 times a day.

9) Phant 3-4 times a day.

- **MSK** 3-4 times a day.

14. Hepatitis (Yakrutvikar)

Introduction :

Inflamation of Liver, Obstruction to passage to bile from liver. Anorexia, debility, fever, heaviness in abdomen, yellow coloured urine, clay coloured stools are symptoms.

1) Guti / Vati (Tablets) :

- **Arogyavardhini** 250-500 mgms with water 3 times a day.
- **Livcom** 2 tablets 3 times a day.
- **KK tablets** 2 tablets 3 times a day.
- **Heerakbhasma** tablets 1 tablet 2-3 times a day.
- **Hemagarbha** tablet 1-7 tablet 2-3 times a day.

2) Asava (Medicated wines) :

- **Kumari Asav** 10-20 ml. with water 2 times a day.
- **Kumari kalpa** 10-20 ml. with water after food 2 times a day.

3) Arishta (Medicated wines) :

- **Abhayarishta** 10-20 ml. with water after food, 2 times a day.

4) Paka (Candu) :

- **Kandarapa Pak** 5-10 gms with milk 2 times a day.

5) Snehana (Oil) :

- **Caster oil** 20-50 ml. with water.

6) Phant (Tea)

- **HSG** 2-3 times a day.

15. Skin Disorders (Twakvikara)

Introduction :

Various types of skin disorders are observed. Pruritus, dry or oozing, discoloration or pigmentation, burning and many others are the symptoms.

1) Choorna (Powders) :

- **Nimbgandhak choorna** 250-500 mgms with honey 2 times a day.
- **Panchnimb churna** 250-500 mgms with honey 3 times a day.

2) Guti/Vati (Tablets) :

- **Gandhak rasayan** 500 mgms to 1 gm with honey 3 times a day.
- **Tab. DC** - 1 tablet 3 times
- **Sookshma Triphala** 2 tablets 2-3 times a day.

3) Asava (Medicated wines) :

- **Sarivadyasava** 10-20 ml. with water 2-3 times a day after food.

4) Arishta (Medicated wines) :

- **Khadirarishta** 10-20 ml. with water 3 times a day after meals.

5) Kwatha (decoction) :

- **Mahamanjishthadi kwatha** 20-40 ml. with water 2-3 times a day.

6) Avaleha (Jam) :

- **Bhallatakavleha** 5-10 ml with milk 2 times a day.
- **Lashunpak** 5-10 mll milk with 2-3 time a day.

7) Tail (Oil) :

- **Paribhadra tail** - external application 1-2 times a day.

- **Vranashodhan Tail** - external application once a day.

7) Ghruta (Ghee) :

- **Shatadhatughruta** - external application 1-2 times a day.

8) Bhasma (Cal x Ash) :

- **Suvarnaraj Vangeshwar** 50-125 mgms with honey or water 3 times a day.
- **Vangbhasma** 250-500 mgms with honey or milk 3 times a day.

9) Ahar (Diet/Food) :

- Avoid sour, salty, pungent food.

10) Phant (Tea)

- **DC** 2-3 times a day.

16. Vommiting (Chhardi)

Introduction :

It is a symptom in many diseases. Half digested food along with water is coming up & out through moutn.

1) Choorna (Powders)

- **Eladi choorna** 1-3 gms. with honey two to four times a day.

2) Guti / Vati (Tablets) :

- **Suvarna sootashekhar** 250 mgms 2-3 times a day with lemon juice or ginger juice.
- **Anticol** 2 tablets 3 times a day.
- **Bruhatvata chintamani** 25-50 mgm with honey

or ginger juice lick repeatedly.

3) Bhasma (Calx = Ash)

- **Kapardik Bhasma** 250-500 mgms with lemon juice, buttermilk or honey 3 times a day.
- **Shankh Bhasma** - 500 mgms to 1 gm. with honey or lemon juice 3 times a day.
- **Jahar mohara pishti** 250 mgms to 500 mgms with honey 3 times a day.
- **Mayurpichamashi** 250-500 mgm with honey four times a day.

10

Appendix

A) Baal Rogi Pariksha Vidhi
(Examination of the Patient)

1) Trividha Pariksha (Three folded examination) :

1) Darshan (Observation)

2) Sparshan (Palpation)

3) Prashna (Questionaries)

All these three have their own importance.

2) Ashtavidha Pariksha (Eight folded examination):

a) Nadi - Pulse - for its speed, strength, type (Sarpa/ Manduk or Hansa)

b) Mala - Stool exam. for 'amata' and 'Krumi' (parasites) etc.

c) Mutra - Urine examination.

d) Jivha - Tongue examination - gives an idea about digestion and annavaha strotas.

e) Druk - eye - sight - eye examination.

f) Sparsha - Temparature, hard or softness - hot/ cold boils or palpatory method.

g) Shabda - Sounds are differentiated of thoracic/ cardiac, peristaltic movements, abdominal - distentions or others.

h) Akruti - Constitution or natural structure of the body.

3) Dashvidha exam (Ten foldea examination) :

a) Dushya - Affected dhatu or mal - is said to be dushya, Such as - Rakta is dushya and pitta is dosha in 'Raktapitta'

b) Desh - Geographical place where disease takes place or part of the body.

c) Bala - Strength of the body.

d) Kala - Time factor in all aspects.

e) Agni - Appetite or digestive power.

f) Prakruti - Constitution of individual.

g) Vaya - Age factor.

h) Satwa - Capability to bare the physical/mental tension of the disease.

i) Satmya - Suitable to body, by nature.

j) Ahar - diet.

According to these 10 points 'avastha' - condition of the disease - changes - So as the 'diagnosis', is achieved.

B) Principles of Treatment According to Doshas

VATA :

i) Oliation (Sneha)
ii) Sweating (Sweda)
iii) Mild laxative (Mrudu Samshodhana)
iv) Sweet, Sour, Salty and hot food, drink and medicines
v) Oil application followed by bath
vi) Body Massage

PITTA :

i) Ghee-intake
ii) Sweet and cold, Purgation
iii) Sweet, Pungent, Astringent food articles and Medicine.

KAPHA :

i) Strong Purgatives
ii) Strong vomiting
iii) Dry and less quantity of food
iv) Strong and hot food
v) Pungent, bitter astringent food articles

B) Therapeutic Index

Disease / Symptom	Medicine	Disease / Symptom	Medicine
Acidity	Pittashamak		
Abortion (Habitual)	Garbhapal Ras	Debility	chyavanprasha
Anaemia	Raktavardhak Tapyadilohavati, Lohassva, Ferite	Diabetes Dysentery	Asanad Kutaj Parpati Vati
		Dyspepsia	Shankha vati
Appetite (To Stimulate)	Panchakolasava Livcom	Dysurea	Gokshuradi Guggul, Varunadi Tablets
		Expectorant	Kantakari Kalp
Ascites	Kumari Asav	Fatigue	Shatavari Kalp
Asthma	Swaskuthar	Fever	Tribhuvan kirti, chandrakala
Cellulitis	Sookshma triphala	Growth (Promoter)	Calcipral
Colds	Parijatak Guti		
Colic (Abdominal)	Lashunadi Vati	Hyperacidity	Calciprite
Constipation	Sukhasarak Choorna / vati		
Convalescence	Raktavardhak, Gold Compound		
Cough	Vasosin, Sitopaladi choorna		
Dermatological disorders	Thiostanin	Diarrhoea	Shankhodar, Kutajarishta, Kurchico
		Flatulence	Charcosal

Indigestion	Amex	Rheumatism	Punarnava Guggul
Jaundice	Kumari Kalp		
Kidney Stone	Varunadi quath		
Laryngitis	Cozenges		
Liver disorders Uishirasava	Arogya Vardhini	Urinary infection	
		Urticaria	Sarivadyasava
Menstrual irregular	Saraswatarishta	Worm infestation	Wormol, Vidangarishta Krumimudgar ras Krumikuthar rasa
Nervine Weakness	Prasham		
Obesity	Kumbhajatu Triphala guggulu		
Oedema	Punarnavasava		
Oral hygiene	Rasadanti		
Pruritus	Thiostanin		
Respiratory Infection	Kanakasava, Suvarna, Malini Vasant		

(Ayurveda Rasashala, Pune. INDIA)

C) A concept of "Ayurvedic - Astrology" related to Mother-Care & Baby-Care

Ayurvedic - Astrology : Mother's Horoscope will be helping tool to Husband-wife and Doctors as mentioned below.

1) Advice about Primary/Secondary sterility - Infertility status.
2) Advice about Ideal Days, Months, Year for conception and better results.
3) Help to monitor Monthly foetus-development in pregnancy (Reference given below).
4) Help to select Medicine - Rasayanas, Panchkarma, Diet - Aahar-vihar, Rutucharya - Seasonal conducts, Yogasana etc. by knowing weak srotas and planet's periods (Mahadasha).
5) Help to know Date of child delivery by mother's horoscope.
6) Help to know probable type delivery - Normal or Operative manner.

Monthly foetus development has been mentioned by Ancient Astrologer Varah Mihir in his books of Ayurvedic Medical Astrology - Bhruhat Jatak Samhita, Jatakadeshmarga as follows -

कललघनां कुरास्थि चर्मांगजचेतनताः । सितकुजजीवसूर्य चंद्रार्किबुधाः परतः ।।
उदयपतिचंद्रसूर्य नाथाः क्रमशोगदिता । भवति शुभाशुभं च मासाधिपतेः सदृशं ।।

बृहत्जातक = निकेषाध्याय ४:१६

Month of Pregnancy	Foetus Status	Lord of Month
1st Month	Kalal	Sukra/Venus
2nd	Ghana (Sukra+Shonit)	Mangal/Mars
3rd	Ankur	Guru/Jupiter
4th	Asthi/Bones	Ravi/Sun
5th	Charma/Skin	Chandra/Moon
6th	Nakh-lome (Nail-Hair)	Shani/Saturn
7th	Chetna/Liveness	Budh/Mercury
8th	Aadhan Lagna	A Lagna Lord
9th	--	Chandra/Moon
10th	--	Ravi/Sun

Meaning by - As per the Status of the Monthly Planetery Lord indicates - Status about monthly foetal developments. According to that medicines to mother for a healthy and inteligent Baby may be advised.

There are 16 Sanskaras - Following two are benificial to Mother and her Child.

1) Garbha Dana - 2 hrs. Muhurta (Span of Time) calculated from the Horoscopes of healthy Mother and Father. Between two Mother's Horoscope is important. She should be healthy by body and mind - during and after the Pregnancy.

2) Pusanvan Vidhi (Desired Progeny) - In 1 to 3rd Months of pregancy. In which pregnant Mother's Health and Psychology (Aahar-Vihar-Vichar) is treated by Ayurveda and Astrology. In this - Diet - Medicine - Reading of riligious prayers - Books etc. are advised.

Dr. Shrikant N. Bhide (I.I.M.)

11

Research References

A) Institute for Post Graduate Teaching & Research In Ayurved, Jamnagar

1) *Stanya* – Raval K.M. – 1973 – M.D.

2) Balakon Men Kaphaja *Krimi* – Solanki S.S. – 1974 – M.D.

3) *Datodbheda* – Janya Vyadhi – Pathak S.D. – 1975 – M.D.

4) *Balatisar* – Kothri R.V. – 1976 – M.D.

5) *Balashosha* – Damania P.J. – 1976 – M.D.

6) A study on the relationship of Foetal *heart rate* with that of the maternal heart rate – Kulkarni K.K. – 1977 – M.D.

7) How a child *differs* from an adult – Chauhan V.S. – 1977

8) Effect of *Jambu* on the *growth pattern* of young rats – Panigrahi M. – 1977 – M.D.

9) Certain aspects of study on *physical growth* – Trivedi A.R. – 1981 – M.D.

10) Response of the New Born to *Madhu Ghrita* – Kamath M.S. – 1981 – M.D.

11) Effect of certain Ayurvedic drug compounds on *pravahika* – (Ms.) Patel S.C. – 1981 - M.D.

12) Effect of Bhumyamalaki in *Jwaras* (with special reference to Vishamajvara) – Kishan T. – 1982 – M.D.

13) Effect of Bhumyamalaki on *Hepato-spleenomegaly* (Yakrut- pleeha vriddhi) – Vora A.C. – 1982 – M.D.

14) Effect of Bhumyamalaki on gastric secretion with special reference to the concept of *Mandagni* – Bhatt M.J. – 1982 – M.D.

15) A study on *growth & development* of infants in Jamnagar – Thakar Bala – 1983 – M.D.

16) *Anabolic effect* of certain Ayurvedic drugs in infancy and childhood – Shastri Krishna M. – 1983 – M.D.

17) A study on the effect on an indigenous drug on *Atisara* – Ramesh Babu L – 1983 – M.D.

18) A study on effect of certain indigenous drug in *Vishamajvara* – Kashaih M. – 1983 – M.D.

19) A study on *Apakarshna of Krimis* (with special reference to Nematodes in the gut) – Suthar M.N. – 1983 – M.D.

20) Response of *Leukocytosis* of an indigenous drug compound – Krishnaiha N – 1983 – M.D.

21) Study of Vitiated *breast milk* as an etiological factor in paediatric disorders - Jagyasi S.N. – 1983 – M.D.

22) A study on the effect of Kata Taila Basti in *Purishaja Krimi* in children below twelve years (with special reference to Enterobius Vevmicularis) – Ramchandran S.K. – 1984 – M.D.

23) Influence of *Chaturbija* on certain Vatika diseases in the field of Kaumarbhritya – Munoli B.T. – 1984 – M.D.

24) *Stanya Kshaya* – ek Adhyayan – (Ms.) Parekh D.T. – 1984 – M.D.

25) *Brimhana (Anabolic)* effect of certain Ayurvedic drugs compound in under weight child – 1985 - Patel K.S. – MD.

26) Role of *Puyaharayoga* in paediatric *skin infections* (Pyogenic) – 1985 – Gohel Jayant S. – M.D.

27) Survey on *growth* and development of infants in Jamnagar 1985 – Thaker Bala p.

28) A survey of *nutritional status* in children based on Ayurvedic concept – 1986 – Sharma Surender – M.D.

29) Effect of certain indigenous drugs in *Purishaja Krimi* – 1986 – Trivedi Y.D. – M.D.

30) Study of *Prakriti* in new born based on psychosomatic considerations – 1986 – Upadyaya – M.D.

31) Role of certain indigenous drugs on *chhardi* in kaumarbritya practice – 1986 – Uma T.K. – M.D.

32) A study on *satva* (mental constitution) in school going children of jamnagar – 1987 – Chacko P.T. – M.D.

33) The role and prevention of *Vighata* in shariravriddhi in children – 1987 – Pune Ashoka B. – M.D.

34) *Brimhana (Anabolic)* effect of certain indigenous drugs in pediatric practice – 1987 – Sharma Chamanlal – M.D.

35) A comparative study of syrup preperation in the management of *Balatisara.* 1988-Shah K.M. – M.D.

36) Studies on the phenomenon of Vyadhikshamatva with special reference to Immunogenicity by using certain *Balya Beans* in experimental animals and Neonates. 1989-Rao A.R.

37) A study of *Bala pakshaghata (Poliomyelitis)* with special reference to its management in practice using certain indigenous drugs and panchakarma procedure. 1990-Kurikala Ashok Kumar-M.D.

38) Studies on mentally retarded children and its management by certain *Medhya Drugs.* 1990-Tiwari A.K-M.D.

39) Study on efficacy of Shivamodaka and Yapanabasti in the management of *Balashosha* with special reference to marasmus. 1991-Vyas P.P.-M.D.

40) A clinical srudy on *Shaiyamutra* (Enursis). 1992-Vyas V.P.-M.D.

41) A study on management of *Balatisara* with certain Ayurvedic formulations. 1993- Sharma R-M.D.

42) A clinical study on *Kasa Roga* in child- hood. 1994-Tiwari R.P.-M.D.

43) A clinical study on Yakrit Roga with special reference to *Kamala* in children. 1995-Rajgopal S.-M.D.

44) Role of *medhya Rasayana* in school children. 1996 – Dash P.B. – M.D.

45) Role of *Garbha poshaka yoga* in the new borns administering the drug in 3rd trimester of pregnancy. 1996 – Jaiswal P.J. – M.D.

46) A study on assessment of certain *indigenous Immunoprotective drugs* in growing children. 1994- Ashok Kumar – Ph.D.

47) Screening of certain Indigenous drugs for *Immunogenecity* in experimental animals and evaluation of their role in Yuadhikshamaṭva status of children. 1995- Rao R.A. – Ph.D.

B) Faculty of Ayurveda,
Institute of medical sciences
Banaras Hindu University Varanasi.

48) Effect of *Kanchanar guggulu* and Dashanga lepa on Gaṇdamala in children – 1967 – Dixit S.B. – M.D.

49) Effect of *Lohachikitsa* in Balyoga with special reference to *balashosha* (marasmus) 1968 – Lalit O.P. – M.D.

50) Ayurvedic management of *Kasa Roga* in children 1969 – Mishra K. – M.D.

51) Effect of certain indigenous drugs in *convulsions* in children 1970 – Dixit S.P. – M.D.

52) Clinical and laboratory studies on *Krimi Roga* in children 1971 – Nand S. – M.D.

53) Experimental & clinical studies on *Balarasayana* 1971 – Devanath P.C. – M.D.

54) Role of certain indigenous drugs in *H. nana infections* in children 1972 – Sharma R.D. – M.D.

55) Studies on Balagrahas with special reference to mukha mandika *(Indian childhood ciurhosis)* 1972 – Shastri C.H.S. – M.D.

56) Clinical & experimental trail of certain indigenous drugs in childhood *anaemia* 1973 – Mishra D.M. – M.D.

57) Effect of certain indigenous drugs in *eosinophilia* in children 1973 – Sahu R.B. – M.D.

58) Erradication of *Ascarias lumbricoides* infestation by certain indigenous drugs in children 1975 – Pandey R.V. – M.D.

59) EFFECT OF Hedychium spicatum in paediatrics tropical pulmonary *eosinophilia* 1975 – Sharma K.L. – M.D.

60) Effect of *Kutaj* Cholerhena antidysentrica on childhood giardiasis 1976 – Tewari Gopal – M.D.

61) Treatment of *Ascariasis* in children with sinduwara (vitex nirgundo Linn) 1978 – Jha K.M. – M.D.

62) Effect of dadima chatussama in *balatisara* – 1981 – Hari Shankar – M.D.

63) Contribution of *Kashyapa Samhita* in paediatrics 1982 – Sastry V.L.N. – M.D.

64) Management of *Post-Polio paresis* with certain Ayurvedic recipes 1984- Mahapatra K.B. – M.D.

65) Studies on *Medhya* effect of Asthamangala Ghrita in children 1984 – Abhimanyu Kumar – M.D.

66) Studies on the effect of Vatagajankush Rasa in *post polio parasis* 1985 – Sharma Anil Kumar – M.D.

67) Studies on effect of *Kumarkalyana Avaleha'* on growth & development in child 1987 – Pawar S.R. – M.D.

68) Studies on effect of Kumarkalyan Avaleha in Boarderline *mentally retarded* children 1988 – Sethi Hem Prakash – M.D.

69) Effect of khanjanikar Rasa in *Balapakshaghata* 1989 – Reddy B.V. S. – M.D.

70) Ayurvedic approach to *aseptic care* of new born – 1990 – Swami T.T. – M.D.

71) Role of Basti in the treatment of balapakshaghata *(post polio paresis)* 1991 – Sahu P.K. – M.D.

72) Role of Lehas on Prevention of upper *respiratory infections* in infants 1991 – Chandra Shekhar – M.D.

73) Study of *Balya* effect of Vidanga compound 1992 – Harichandan B.K. – M.D.

74) A study on *immunological aspect* of balarasayana 1975 – Dixit S.P. – M.D.

75) Principles and *practice of paediatrics* in Ayurveda 1977 – Shastry C.H.S. – Ph.D.

76) Studies on *Phakka Roga* including *Balashosha* 1978 – Dixit B.S.- Ph.D.

77) Role of *medhya rasayana* in children 1981 - Sharma R.D. – Ph.D.

78) Studies of *Brimhana effect* of certain Lehas mentioned for children 1987 – Hari shankar – Ph.D.

C) National Institute of Ayurveda Rajasthan Uiversity, Jaipur.

79) Balakon men *krimi Roga* Evam Mustadi yoga ka Chikitsatmaka Adhyavan. Kasim M. – 1991 – M.D.

80) *Balatisara* men Bilvadi Yoga ka chikitsatmaka Adhyayan. Sharma N. – 1991 – M.D.

81) *Dantodbhava* Vyapada Evam kashyapa Ghrita chikitsatmaka Adhyayan. 1992 – Rai D.K. – M.D.

82) Balyavastha men *kasa roga* ke pariprekshya men kasaghna yoga ki karmukta. 1992 – Sharma S.K. – M.D.

83) *Bala shosha* Roga men Bala shoshahar Rasayan ka chikitsatmaka Adhyayan. 1992 – Sharma R. – M.D.

84) Balakon ke Tundikevi ke Pariprekshya men *Pitaka Yoga* ka prabhavatmaka Adhyayan. 1993 – Shama Sudhakar. – M.D.

85) Balakon men Yakriddalyudar Par *Guda Pippali* ka chikitsatmak Adhyayan. 1994 – (Smt.) Kaur Manjit. – M.D.

86) Koumarbhritya ke pariprekshya men *Kashyapa samhita* ; Ek Adhyayan – 1994 – Singh A.K. – M.D.

87) *Bala Pakshaghat* men Mahanarayan Taila ki karmukata (Matra Basti ke pariprekshya men) – Jain C.M. – M.D.

88) *Dantodbhed* kalin vyadiyon men dantodbheda Gadantaka Rasa ka prabhavotmaka Adhyayan – 1994 – Agrawal A. K. – M.D.

89) *Maha Pishachik Ghrita* ke bala naganga vriddhikar Bava ka Adhyayan – 1995 – Mishra V.K. – M.D.

90) Tina se Dasha varsha vaya-varga vishesha ke balakon men *vriddhi Evam vikas* (Sharir ka Ayam) ka ayurvediya pariprekshaya – Jain R.K. – M.D.

91) Shashtrokta *Guduchyadi Rasayan* ke medhya prabhava Balakon men : Ek Adhyayan – 1995 – Satthu (Ms.) S. – M.D.

92) Balakon men sutrakrimi par *shigru* Aur *Akhukarni* ke chikitsatmak prabhava ka Tulanatmak Adhyayan – 1995 – Lal N.P. – M.D.

93) Katipaya Rasa Bhaishjya kalpanaon ki *Balshosha* men Karmukata (madhumalini Vasant, Ashvagandha Evam Katuka kalpa ke pariprekshya men) – 1992 – Jain C.M. Ph.D.

D) Rajasthana University Jaipur M.M.M. Govt. Ayurvedic College, Udaipur.

94) *Bala pakshaghata* : Ek Ayurvediya Nidana Chikitsatmaka Adhyayan – 1984 – Sharma Loknath. – Ph.D. Thesis

E) Pune University, Pune.

95) Studies of Bala Pakshaghata *(Poliomyelities)* & its management by Panchkarma Therapy – Yadeyaha P. – Ph.D. University of Pune Ph.D. Thesis

F) Post graduate Research Project - Institute of Indian Medicine, Pune.

96) Sycora & *Paediatric Cough* - Dr. Kshama Vaidya (IIM) 1988

97) Use of Baljeevan in *child health Care* - Dr. J.K. Barde 1995

98) Use of Nasya & Abhayanga in *cerebral palsy* - Dr. D.J. Khasgiwale 2000

99) Efficacy of Krumimodgar Rasa *Purishja Krumi* - Dr. V. D. Sathe 1999

100) Role of Ashwagandha Shatavari as tab on *foetal & maternal health* during antenatal care - Dr. Manjiri Deshpande. 1999

101) Study of effect of Prasham & Brahmiprash in the management of *Hyperactive Children* – Dr. Pramod Bankhele. I.I.M. 1997

102) Use of Prasham on *mentally retarded children* – Vd. Rajendra Pawar. I.I.M. 1998

103) *Shayyamutra* (Bed wetting) - Dr. P.A. Suru I.I.M. 1994

104) Sanjeevani Vati & *diarrhoea in children.* – Dr. (Mrs.) Belgamwar. I.I.M. 1996

105) Clinical evaluation of wormol in paediatrics with special reference to *intestinal worms* – Nanal Hospital / AR / Dr. Yogesh Bendale. 1996

105) Obesity in school children A sample survey of schools of Pune - Dr. P. V. Paranjpe - 1994

107) Krumimudgar Rasa & psoriasis - Dr. D. J. Khasgiwale - 1998

108) Clinical study of Bramiprash Ghan in mental fatigue - Dr. B.B. Date - 1997

109) Use of Sanjeevani Guti in Atisar - Dr. A. R. Shitre - 1996

12

Bibliography

1) Marathi Charak Samhita - Dr. P. H. Kulkarni - Sagar Prakashan - 1982

2) Marathi Sushrut Samhita - Dr. P. H. Kulkarni - Sagar Prakashan - 1985

3) Dr. P. H. Kulkarni's Ayurveda Research Papers - Dr. B. B. Date - Ayurveda Rasashala - 1999

4) Ayurveda Therapy - Dr. P. H. Kulkarni - Ayurveda Rasashala - 1997

5) Ayurveda Aahara - Dr. P. H. Kulkarni - Ayurveda Education Series - 1998

6) Handbook of Clinical Ayurveda Practice - Dr. P. H. Kulkarni - Ayurveda Education Series - 1999

7) Lecture Notes - Intensive Teaching Programme for Foreign Students - 1988, 1991, 1993 and 1996 - Institute of Indian Medicine.

8) Deerghayu International - Vol. I & XVII - 1984-2000

Our Other Titles on Ayurveda and Herbal Medicine

The Ayurveda Encyclopaedia: Natural Secrets to Healing, Prevention & Longevity/Swami Sada Shiva Tirtha

The Caraka Samhita-English Translation/A.C. Kaviratna, Ed. And Revised by P. Sharma, 5 Vols.

Secrets of Ayurvedic Massage/ Atreya Smith

Ayurveda Ahar (Food / Diet) / P. H. Kulkarni

Bronchial Asthma Care in Ayurveda and Holistic Systems/ P. H. Kulkarni

Joint Disorders Care in Ayurveda / P. H. Kulkarni

Ayurvedic Clinical Medicine/ A. Vinaya Kumar

Heartcare in Ayurveda / P. H. Kulkarni

Handbook of Clinical Ayurveda Practice / P. H. Kulkarni

Ayurveda Therapy/ P.H. Kulkarni

Ayurveda Herbs/ P.H.Kulkarni

Ayurveda Minerals/ P.H.Kulkarni

Ayurveda Panchakarma/ P.H.Kulkarni

Secret Potions, Elixirs & Concoctions/ Marie Anakee Miczak

Herbal First Aid and Health Care/ Kyle D. Christensen

Fundamentals of Ayurvedic Medicine (Revised & Enlarged Edition) / Vaidya Bhagwan Dash

Encyclopaedia of Domestic Medicine/Thomas J. Graham

Clinical Application of Ayurvedic Remedies and a List of Ayurvedic Preparations

Uncommon Plant Drugs of Ayurveda/Gyanandra Pandey

Pharmacopoeial Standards of Herbal Plants/C.R. Karnick

Medicinal Plants of Himalayas/Gyanendra Pandey

The Natural Remedy Book for Women/Diane Stein

The Male Herbal: Health Care for Men and Boys/James Green

A Glossary of Ayurveda, Tibetan & Unani Medicines

A Comparative Study of Ayurveda and Treatment by Indian Drugs/P.K. Chitale